The Structure of the Retina

The Structure of the Retina

By

SANTIAGO RAMÓN Y CAJAL

Late Professor of Histology and Pathology
Faculty of Medicine
University of Madrid
Madrid, Spain

Compiled and Translated by

Sylvia A. Thorpe, Sc.M.

Walter S. Hunter Laboratory of Psychology
Brown University
Providence, Rhode Island

and

Mitchell Glickstein, Ph.D.

Walter S. Hunter Laboratory of Psychology
Brown University
Providence, Rhode Island

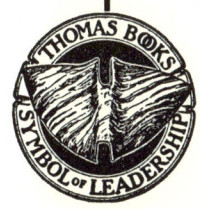

CHARLES C THOMAS • PUBLISHER
Springfield • Illinois • U.S.A.

Published and Distributed Throughout the World by
CHARLES C THOMAS • PUBLISHER
BANNERSTONE HOUSE
301-327 East Lawrence Avenue, Springfield, Illinois, U.S.A.
NATCHEZ PLANTATION HOUSE
735 North Atlantic Boulevard, Fort Lauderdale, Florida, U.S.A.

This book is protected by copyright. No part of it may be reproduced in any manner without written permission from the publisher.

© *1972, by* CHARLES C THOMAS • PUBLISHER
ISBN 0-398-02385-9
Library of Congress Catalog Card Number: 70-175083

With THOMAS BOOKS *careful attention is given to all details of manufacturing and design. It is the Publisher's desire to present books that are satisfactory as to their physical qualities and artistic possibilities and appropriate for their particular use.* THOMAS BOOKS *will be true to those laws of quality that assure a good name and good will.*

Printed in the United States of America
C-1

TRANSLATORS' FOREWORD TO THE ENGLISH EDITION

RAMÓN Y CAJAL'S monograph on the structure of the vertebrate retina was first published in 1892 in the French journal *La Cellule*.[1] Cajal was especially motivated to write this volume because many workers did not have access to, or were unable to read, his earlier reports in Spanish. The work was quickly translated into German by Richard Greeff, and that edition appeared two years later.[2] Finally, in 1933 an updated version of the 1894 edition was published in French.[3] Both revisions of the original monograph contain important additions made by Cajal in the chapters on the avian retina, the development of the retina, the fovea centralis, and the centrifugal fibers. All three editions have been incorporated in our English translation.

The terminology used in the present volume requires some explanation. In some cases we have translated literally, retaining the terms "axis cylinder" and "protoplasmic processes" for the basic extensions of the nerve cell. The reader can circumvent a good deal of historical controversy by thinking of these as "axon" and "dendrite," respectively. In other cases, however, we have selected more modern English terms. For example, Cajal's "cônes jumeaux" ("Zwillingszapfen") are the paired cones found in amphibia, reptiles, and birds; we have translated these as "double cones." In contrast is the "*twin* cone," or cone pair, composed of two identical members fused along their inner segments and found only in teleost fish. Cajal himself clarified the question of the kinds of cells which can be found on the vitreous side of the inner nuclear layer. He used the older term "spongioblast" for those cells of the inner nuclear layer which have an axis cylinder in the optic nerve. He also coined the term "amacrine cell" to refer to those cells in the same retinal layer which do *not* have an axis cylinder.

In the present volume Cajal gives a detailed description of all

v

types of retinal cells in representatives of each vertebrate class, together with an account of the way in which these cells are interconnected. By using the Golgi staining method, which stains but a few cells with all their processes, he could see and describe in detail the shape of the retinal cells and the course and distribution of their fine processes. From these observations he was able to reconstruct the arrangement of retinal cells and describe the pattern in which they appeared to be connected to one another.

Ramón y Cajal's retinal studies are an anatomical masterpiece, but at the time he wrote, physiological concepts and techniques were insufficient for functional analysis of the structure and interconnections he described. Cajal himself could only speculate on the functions of retinal cells and the possible meaning of their connections. While his speculations are often imaginative, they are limited by his somewhat oversimplified view of synaptic mechanisms. For example, nowhere in this volume does he interpret synapses as doing anything other than exciting the next neuron in the pathway.

In recent years physiological analysis has progressed to the point where it can now make more complete use of Cajal's detailed descriptions of the retina. A major step in this direction was the development of the idea of a receptive field and the application of single-unit recording to retinal ganglion cells.[4] In most ganglion cells illumination of some small part of the visual field increases the firing rate, while illumination of a nearby region will decrease it. The area in which light will excite the cell, combined with the area in which light will inhibit the cell, is termed the "receptive field." Given such a concept, we are in a position to ask an analytical question: How does information from the photoreceptors reach the ganglion cells to produce the observed receptive fields? Clearly, detailed knowledge of the types of cells in the retina and their mode of interconnection is a prerequisite to answering such a question.

Many retinal elements do not fire action potentials; hence, physiological analysis using only extracellular recording must be incomplete. With the introduction of intracellular recording, however, it is now possible to analyze the responses of cells which produce only graded potentials. For example, the spectral sensitivity of individual cones can be specified by recording directly the receptor potential in response to different wavelengths of light.[5] Furthermore, by studying the potential recorded intracellularly from cells in the inner nuclear layer,[6] some understanding of the interconnections between retinal cell types, and thus of the construction of receptive fields, can be gained. Cajal's contributions to retinal anatomy are essential to these recent electrophysiological studies.

Basically, Cajal describes the retina as a structure composed of three layers of cells, the processes of which connect with one another in two plexiform layers. In teleost fish and mammals, where the knobby rod termination is clearly distinguishable from the filamentous cone termination, he contrasts bipolar cells which contact the cones with bipolar cells which contact the rods; these bipolars in turn make preferential contact with distinct ganglion cells. Cajal thus proposes a rod pathway and a cone pathway through the retina, each being relatively isolated from the other. However, some ganglion cells contact *both* types of bipolar cells, suggesting that rod and cone information can be shared. Physiologists have provided definite evidence that rods and cones may be functionally connected to the same ganglion cell, but the extent of independence and of convergence in these two pathways remains to be learned.

The inner nuclear layer contains several cell types. In addition to the bipolar cells, there are the horizontal cells, the amacrine cells, and the nuclei of the Müller fibers. Cajal suggested functional roles for these cells which may be established and extended by current workers. For example, the shape and extent of the Müller fibers suggested a role in the support of other retinal elements and isolation of their conduction paths through the retina. His description of the horizontal cells and their processes provides an excellent background for understanding their probable role in the construction of receptive fields. Cajal himself proposed that these elements might serve to bring various groups of receptors in relation to one another. The structure and connections of the amacrine cells pose equally fascinating problems for fundamental study. Not only do these cells have no axon, but also their processes are arranged in a very particular manner. The dendritic trees of the ganglion cells spread at different levels within the inner plexiform layer and form associations with the processes of the amacrine and bipolar cell processes, thereby creating the distinct laminar appearance of this layer so clearly described by Cajal.

An obvious question arises for physiological study: Are there unique receptive field properties associated with ganglion cells whose processes extend into different sublayers of the inner plexiform layer? Intracellular recording and dye-marking techniques provide the tools to answer this important question.

Cajal discusses two types of connections in the retina which serve a possible feedback role: the centrifugal fibers and the Landolt clubs. The centrifugal fibers are especially prominent in birds, but their existence in all vertebrates remains in dispute. Landolt clubs, which are found in the amphibian, reptilian, and avian retina, arise from a single ascending branch of a bipolar cell and course through the outer nuclear layer. Analysis of the physiological role of the Landolt clubs and the centrifugal fibers remains an important problem for understanding retinal function.

Cajal was struck by the relative uniformity of the retina across vertebrates. To him specialization of the retina seemed to be related not so much to the animal's phylogenetic status as to the structural characteristics and the relative distribution of rods and cones, and thus to be a function of the visual requirements of the animal. In view of Cajal's comparative insights, it is surprising that only in passing did he mention the photomechanical responses of the photoreceptors and pigment epithelium to light and darkness.

It is clear throughout this volume that Cajal was addressing himself to a fundamental problem of neuroanatomy: that of the interconnections between nerve cells in general. He proposed that nerve impulses were transmitted from cell to cell by means of contact between cell processes. Cajal's views were in direct opposition to the nerve net theory, to which most histologists of that era subscribed. According to the nerve-net theory, nerve processes are fused to form a net or syncytium. Dogiel was one of the most enthusiastic proponents of this theory, and Cajal's rather biting criticisms and comments about him can best be understood in the light of this controversy. Cajal argued that the methylene blue stain used by Dogiel (Ehrlich's method) would not allow one to differentiate between fibers which simply cross one another from those that actually fuse.

In some cases Cajal's faith in the neuron doctrine was sustained even in the face of apparently contradictory evidence. For example a process of a bipolar cell occasionally appeared to fuse with the terminal spherule of a rod, thereby giving the appearance of cells being joined in a kind of syncytium. With the resolution of the electron microscope, we can now interpret this apparent fusion. The bipolar cell process invaginates the rod spherule, along with the horizontal cell processes, so that a special synaptic complex is formed.[7]

It is clear that Ramón y Cajal's work provides the structural basis for many current physiological questions: What is the direct pathway through the retina, and how is it modified by lateral interactions within the plexiform layers to produce the receptive fields of retinal ganglion cells? How are we to interpret functionally the striking lamination of the inner plexiform layer? What is the nature of the feedback connections in the retina, and to what extent are these effected by centrifugal fibers or Landolt clubs?

Even though Ramón y Cajal's investigations were done nearly eighty years ago, they provide a broad and solid base for approaching these fascinating problems. Indeed, in many respects Cajal's studies remain the most outstanding and comprehensive descriptions of retinal structure to date.

Sylvia A. Thorpe
Mitchell Glickstein

REFERENCES

1. Ramón y Cajal, S.: La rétine des vertébrés. *La Cellule*, 1892 (9).
2. Ramón y Cajal, S.: *Die Retina der Wirbeltiere.* (Greeff, R., trans.), Wiesbaden, 1894.
3. Ramón y Cajal, S.: La rétine des vertébrés. *Trav. d. Labor. d. Rech. biol. d. l'Univ. d. Madrid*, 1933 (28).

4. Kuffler, S.: Discharge patterns and functional organization of the mammalian retina. *J. Neurophysiol.*, 1953 (16), 37-68.
5. Tomita, T., Kaneko, A., Murakami, M., and Pautler, E.: Spectral response curves of single cones in the carp. *Vis. Res.*, 1967 (7), 519-531.
6. Werblin, F. and Dowling, J.: Organization of the retina of the mudpuppy, *Necturus maculosus*. II. Intracellular recording. *J. Neurophysiol.*, 1969 (32), 339-355.
7. Dowling, J. and Boycott, B.: Organization of the primate retina: Electron microscopy. *Proc. Royal Soc. London,* 1966 (160), 80-111.

TRANSLATOR'S FOREWORD TO THE GERMAN EDITION

I SPENT a long time at the Senckenberg Pathological-Anatomical Institute in Frankfurt-am-Main learning the Golgi-Cajal chromium-silver method for studying the central nervous system and applying that method to the retina, which is decidedly more difficult. While I was there, I happened upon Ramón y Cajal's great and meaningful work, "The Retina of Vertebrates," in the journal *La Cellule* (1892). When I had read this work—the fruit of Cajal's many years of diligent effort—it seemed most important for me to introduce his writing to German ophthalmology. Cajal reported brilliant new results which exceeded our expectations so greatly, that by comparison my own findings were of negligible value.

The chromium-silver staining method of Golgi has brought about a profound change in the field of neuroanatomy. Although neurologists and anatomists have been busy for the last few years emulating the results of Golgi and Cajal (e.g. Kölliker, His, Waldeyer), these completely new views of the anatomy and physiology of the retina have received little attention from the ophthalmologists. This neglect is probably due to the fact that the relevant publications appeared in Italian (Tartufri) and in Spanish (Cajal); thus they are difficult to understand and to obtain. In addition, training in these new staining techniques demands much time, and they are especially difficult in the retina.

While it is true that this most recent and great work of Ramón y Cajal is published in French, I would like to emphasize that I did not decide to publish this book because I do not credit German scholars with the ability to read French books, but rather for the following reasons: (a) It seemed important to make such a significant work more readily available, since articles appearing in *La Cellule* are not widely circulated in our country.

(In all of Berlin I could procure it only in the Königsbibliotek, and even then the book could not be checked out of the reading room.) (b) I wanted to consider the early Spanish and Italian works, insofar as they were relevant, and to give a short review of the development of the new concepts derived from the new methods (the methylene blue stain of Ehrlich and the chromium-osmium-silver stain of Golgi). (c) I was aware that reading Cajal's French article, especially for those not yet familiar with these methods, is quite difficult. This is especially true because a number of technical terms have no German equivalents as yet, or because they are unfamiliar to readers of either language. Those who have not followed the most recent literature on neuroanatomy are unaware of such terms as "l'épine d'une collaterale," "cellule déplacée," "cellule stratifiée," etc., and thus may not be completely clear on their meaning. The difficulty involved in reading the foreign literature is increased by the large number of newly created terms.

For these reasons the compilation and publication of the present book seemed worthwhile to me. Furthermore, I wanted to bring Cajal's fascinating findings to the attention not only of ophthalmologists but also of a wider scientific circle. According to Cajal, the retina offers the anatomist and neurologist a favorable opportunity for understanding the general morphology of nerve cells and the structure of a nervous center. The recent findings on the retina of different classes of animals should also be welcomed by both the anatomist and the zoologist. Finally, a number of Cajal's highly ingenious hypotheses will be of great interest to the physiologist. Some of them are, to be sure, not yet well established and require empirical verification.

The book contains mainly Ramón y Cajal's studies of the retina which appeared in *La Cellule,* Vol. 9, No. 1 (1892), and also findings from his earlier Spanish and French publications, insofar as they complement the present volume. *These are accompanied by a number of Cajal's latest findings on the retina which have not yet been published;* they are based on recent studies and were kindly sent to me by Professor Ramón y Cajal for translation and inclusion in this book. They occur mainly in the sections entitled "The Retina of Birds," "The Development of

Translator's Foreword to the German Edition xiii

the Retinal Cells," "The Fovea Centralis," etc. The present volume, therefore, is to be regarded for the most part as Ramón y Cajal's original work. The seven plates which are included contain only Cajal's original figures from the 1892 *La Cellule*.

Regarding the translation, I would like to say that I have tried to translate as literally as possible and to remain as close as possible to the phrases of the original text. Perhaps the style has suffered here and there because of this. I have usually used the same word for the recurring names of cellular extensions and nerve endings (e.g. "panache," "arborization," "épine," etc.), and when they are used for the first time, I have often included the names which Cajal used.

Where possible, I have tried to determine which of Cajal's new designations have been used in the recent Spanish and French neuroanatomical literature and carried over into German. Such expressions have been retained, and for technical terms requiring a new translation, I have added Cajal's original term in quotes. I have also added a short explanation when it seemed necessary for understanding the term.

My own opinions are, of course, not intermingled in this work; everything refers strictly to Cajal. Thus, the words "I," "my investigations," etc. refer to him and not to me. Sometimes a brief clarification or a reference to recent literature seemed desirable to me, and the resulting additions are footnotes designated as "Greeff's note."

I am grateful to Professor Ramón y Cajal for his permission to publish this book and especially for sending his valuable new findings for inclusion here. I also thank Professor Carnoy, the publisher of *La Cellule*, who allowed me to use Cajal's text and figures. I would also like to thank Dr. Edinger in Frankfurt-am-Main, who introduced me to Cajal's technique, and Professor Weigert, who gave me a position in his institute.

Even if some of the details of Cajal's findings concerning the structure of the retina are still controversial (c.f. Dogiel's opinions), as a whole they should be regarded as proven and acknowledged by most eminent anatomists. A publication of Cajal's views is timely for the clarification of such controversial questions. It would make me very happy if this book could stimulate appreciation for and interest in Cajal's work, which in the future will probably be regarded as a major contribution to our knowledge of retinal structure.

RICHARD GREEFF

Berlin
March 1894

INTRODUCTION AND REVIEW OF THE LITERATURE

Richard Greeff

THE great change which has recently taken place in our knowledge of the structure of the peripheral and central nervous systems is apparent when the latest journals and textbooks dealing with this matter are compared with those which were written only a few years ago. Many formerly unsolved problems were explained by the use of a special staining and research technique with a property previously unknown and unimagined. In many respects it has advanced our knowledge of the structure and function of the nervous system beyond all hopes and expectations, while simultaneously introducing an entirely new and broad perspective into the field.

After the old carmine staining methods of Grenarcher, Gerlach, and others had been fully exploited by a number of studies, some further progress was made with the classical Weigert hematoxylin method, especially in the pathological and experimental domain. Then there was a very slow advance, or perhaps even a complete standstill, until the latest methods, especially those associated with Ehrlich, Golgi, and Ramón y Cajal, brought us extraordinary success. This change is most striking to someone not immersed in the details of this specialized area of anatomical research when he examines the recent editions of earlier textbooks. Just how much the Golgi-Cajal method has surpassed everything previously known is most apparent after reading the chapter entitled "The Nervous System" in the newly published handbook of Kölliker.[1] The text and figures are constantly based on the authority and words of these two investigators. This can also be noted in the well-written and lucid *Lectures on the Structure of the Central Nervous System* by L. Edinger (4th edition) and other textbooks. In addition to Kölliker, many of our most eminent anatomists and other investigators have been concerned with the work of Golgi and Cajal. I recommend especially the following works, which will serve as an introduction to the new techniques and viewpoints:

> Waldeyer, W.: Über einige neuere Forschungen im Gebiete der Anatomie des Nervensystems. *Deutsch. med. Wochenschr.*, 1891, No. 44, ff.
>
> His, W.: Über den Aufbau unseres Nervensystems. Lecture given at the German Scientific Research meetings in Nürnberg, 1892, Leipzig, 1893, and published in *Berliner klin. Wochenschr.*, 1893 (30), 957.

Both these articles are concerned mainly with the studies of Golgi and Cajal, and express unreserved appreciation and recognition. Other works worth mentioning are the following:

> Kölliker, A.: Eröffnungsrede auf der fünften Versammlung der Anat. Gesellschaft, 1891. *Anat. Anz.*, 1891 (Jahrg. VI).
>
> van Gehuchten, A.: Les decouvertes récentes dans l'anatomie et l'histologie du systeme nerveux général. *Ann. d. l. soc. belg. d. mikros.*, 1891 (15), 113.
>
> van Gehuchten, A.: *Le systeme nerveux de l'homme.* Sierre, 1893.
>
> Retzius, G.: Biologische Untersuchungen. *Neue Folge*, 1892 (4).
>
> Ramón y Cajal, S.: Conexión general de los elementos nerviosos. *La medicina práctica*, 1889 (No. 88), p. 341.
>
> Ramón y Cajal, S.: (Translation of the above article.) *Arch. f. Anat. u. Physiol., Anat. Abt.*, 1893.
>
> Riese, H.: Über die Technik der Golgi-schen Schwarzfärbung durch Silbersalze und über die Ereignisse derselben. *Centralbl. f. path. Anat.*, 1891.
>
> von Lenhossék, M.: Neuere Forschungen über den feineren Bau des Nervensystems. *Correspondensbl. f. Schweiz. Ärzte*, 1891 (Jahrg. 21), p. 489.
>
> von Lenhossék, M.: Der feinere Bau des Nervensystems im Lichte neuester Forschung. *Fortschr. d. Med.*, 1892 (10).

The last work in particular describes the technique and results obtained with it very thoroughly, and also gives a complete review of the literature in which a number of relevant works are cited.

It is worth the effort to review briefly the origins and history of the new methods which are of special significance not only for histological technique but also for understanding the innervation of organs and of cell morphology. Both methods,

Introduction and Review of the Literature   xvii

which became known almost simultaneously (the osmium-dichromate-silver stain of Golgi and the methylene blue stain of Ehrlich for living tissue), are fundamentally different in their application and technique. They are remarkably similar, however, in their effects on the tissue. Both methods have the single, incomparable, and hitherto completely unknown characteristic that they do not uniformly stain all the cells in a section, in contrast to traditional methods. Instead, only isolated cells are stained in the complicated and dense mesh formed by the nerve cells and their processes (e.g. in the cerebellum and the retina), and all of the surrounding cells remain completely spared. Indeed, a single cell can be stained even out to its finest processes. Only in this way is it possible to see the structure of individual nerve cells, which all lie very close to one another. If all these cells and their processes were to stain equally, they would become lost in frightful chaos. The method gives us pictures of previously unimagined beauty and completeness; in thick sections the cells appear almost as if they were drawn schematically. The unusual thickness of the section makes it possible to see cell processes not only at a single plane in a microscopic section but also extending above and below that plane. This property should be quite obvious in the plates accompanying this work. The objection is often made by almost all of my colleagues that such figures must have been made schematically.

The question may be raised as to why only a few cells are impregnated in every case with the silver salts, while other cells of the same section under the same conditions remain completely unstained. At the present time we are not in a position to answer this question unequivocally. However, if we know that the substance must be brought into contact with very fresh, living cells for the stain to be taken up, then we are led to the conclusion that the uptake of the staining material is somehow related to the state of living cells when the organ is placed in the reagent. From this one might suppose that those cells are impregnated, which, at the moment they are placed into the staining solution, happen to be in a particular state of activity, or in a particularly favorable metabolic condition.

The new epoch dates from the discovery of two new methods,

for which we thank Camillo Golgi in Pavia and P. Ehrlich in Berlin. A third person, Ramón y Cajal in Madrid, significantly broadened the application of the Golgi method, improved it, and gave it the great distribution and significance known today throughout the entire scientific world. The first publication of C. Golgi concerning his method and the results obtained with it appeared in the year 1875.[2] At that time, however, the importance of the new method was not yet recognized, and only very slowly did it win acceptance. Golgi's main work appeared in the year 1885.[3] His studies were concerned mainly with the investigation of nervous components in the spinal cord of mature animals. The great change in the method dates mainly from when Cajal began to use it on the central nervous system of young animals and embryos. He showed the scientific world that the most beautiful and clear pictures could be obtained with this method, thereby offering a clearer and simpler account of the nervous system than had ever been imagined. A comprehension of such pictures would give us a schema, so to speak, by which we might be able to understand more complex relations.

Meanwhile in 1886 Ehrlich published his method of staining living nervous tissue with methylene blue.[4] This method is very similar to the Golgi method in its effects on the nerve cell, but its technique and use are completely different. It is an especially fortunate circumstance that the discovery and publication of both methods occurred at approximately the same time. One might have been more justified in his mistrust of the astonishing new methods, and in fact, in many respects it might have remained quite doubtful whether the staining was only accidental silver precipitate or actually the protoplasm of a nerve cell, had it not been possible to control the results obtained with one method by the use of another method which had such different effects on the nerve protoplasm. In point of fact it was found that the results given by both methods were identical in many cases, contrary to the argument that both methods do not give exactly the same picture.

With regard to the methylene blue technique, I refer the reader to numerous descriptions in the German literature (especially those of Ehrlich, Retzius, and Dogiel). I have no personal experience with Ehrlich's method, but an acquaintance with the technique is not absolutely necessary for an understanding of Ramón y Cajal's present work, even though the results obtained with this method are often mentioned. One must know only that when used on living tissue, methylene blue somewhat arbitrarily stains a nerve cell here and there, even out to its finest processes, while sparing the surrounding cells. This action is, of course, just like the chromium-silver stain. The differences which result when using the two methods are often discussed in Cajal's description of the retina.

This is not the place to go into extensive detail about the Golgi-Cajal osmium-dichromate-silver method and the many peculiarities of the production and preservation of the preparations. The most extensive description of such details is given by von Lenhossék in *Fortschritte der Medizin* (1892) and in many of the references cited earlier. Here I intend only to give a very brief description and overview to the reader not yet acquainted with the technique. In general, I would like to say that my introduction does not pretend to offer anything new to the specialist; rather it is meant to bring Cajal's studies on the retina to the attention of the ophthalmologists, who are naturally closest to me, and to those investigators who have not yet had the opportunity to employ the interesting and important new techniques.

Many authors deny the label "method" to the Golgi chromium-silver impregnation technique because it often seems purely accidental whether good staining occurs. One can never be sure of getting a good preparation, and it is almost as if a trick which produces good staining must be discovered for each individual organ or each species. Often when two sections are prepared under the same conditions, one will be well impregnated, and the other, worthless. Sometimes one hundred sections must be prepared without success until one of them, often as if by accident, stains in the desired manner. This single section, however, is so perfect and exquisite that it surpasses anything seen previously, and seems worth all the effort. One must take into account this great capriciousness of the technique. Therefore, a large number of small pieces of the organ to be studied is placed in the first bath; they are gradually removed at different intervals and put into the second bath. Then the individual pieces are examined according to the sequence in which they were treated. If sufficient impregnation has not yet occurred in the sections, they are put back into the first bath, and subsequently, into the second one. Each piece is best numbered in a special small glass container and kept isolated during changing. Often such changing requires several hours, so that the first piece might remain in Bath #1 for twenty-four hours; the second piece, for twenty-five hours, etc. Likewise, the first piece might remain in Bath #2 for twenty-four hours; the second, for twenty-five hours, etc. In this way it may be possible to find a piece of tissue which has remained for neither too long nor too short a time in both baths, and from this piece probably only certain sections will give lovely pictures.

There are three ways to do the Golgi method: the slow method, the mixed method, and the rapid method. I mention these methods only briefly here, as Cajal has already introduced them in his description of the retina. He and most other investigators use the rapid Golgi method almost exclusively. In the slow method the pieces stay some twenty to thirty days in a 2% potassium dichromate solution, and are then put in a 0.75% silver nitrate solution for twenty-four to forty-eight hours. In contrast, in the mixed method the pieces remain four to five days in the first solution and then they are placed for twenty-four to thirty hours in a mixture composed of two parts 1% osmium solution and eight parts 2% potassium dichromate solution; finally, they are put into a 0.75% silver solution for twenty-four to forty-eight hours. The rapid method is described by Cajal in his section, "Investigative Methods," in the present volume. The fresh and almost living pieces are put into osmium dichromate solution, which is composed of one part 1% osmium solution and four parts 3.5% potassium dichromate solution.

The pieces are as small as possible: At the most they are 1 cm^3 but usually not more than 3 or 4 mm on a side. One also cannot be too economical with the solution. On a small (5 mm) piece, about 10 cc of solution or more should be used. (The solution should be freshly prepared.) The pieces remain in this solution twenty-four to forty-eight hours or sometimes longer, and they darken during this time. Afterwards the pieces are dried on filter paper and then put into the second bath, which is composed of 0.75% to 1.0% silver nitrate solution. A brownish cloud of chromium-silver develops immediately in the solution. The pieces remain in this bath about twenty-four hours, or longer if necessary.

The pieces must then be cut immediately and embedded; they are probably hard enough for sectioning without further preparation. However, they may be placed for fifteen minutes in absolute alcohol; a longer exposure to alcohol will cause them to deteriorate. The pieces are then cut between elderberry pulp or pieces of liver, which is very good because the sections can be made very thick (0.7 to 1.0 mm thick). They can also be placed in paraffin immediately, as Cajal has described. I myself have usually embedded sections in celloidin in the following way: The sections are taken from 80% alcohol and put into 100% alcohol for five minutes. Then they are placed in thin celloidin for five minutes. After this, they are covered with thick celloidin for one minute and then dipped into 80% alcohol. Five minutes later sections are made. Every section can be examined immediately for its usefulness under the microscope in alcohol; those which can be used are then taken out of the alcohol and embedded. For this purpose the sections are first placed in absolute alcohol for a very short period of time (one or two minutes), and then in clove oil or mineral oil for the same period of time. A few seconds in xylol are then given to separate the sections from the oil, and they are finally placed in a thin layer of dammar lacquer on a cover glass. To obtain moderately long-lasting preparations it is recommended that the cover slip be placed in the incubator so that the lacquer may dry as fast as possible. The cover glass should not be placed directly on the slide, since exclusion of the air will cause the preparation to deteriorate quickly. For that reason, and also to protect the preparation from dust, two tiny parallel glass rods are glued to the slide so that it is separated from the cover slip by the tips of these rods, with the section underneath. Even with these precautions, sections prepared in this manner do not last a very long time.*

When cutting, if sections are found that are not well impregnated, these are separated from the block, and the pieces (with the accompanying celloidin, if necessary) are put back into the first bath (osmium). The entire procedure is then repeated. (See below: Cajal's double- and triple-impregnation procedures.)

Unfortunately, neither the Golgi stain nor the methylene blue stain are exclusively nerve stains. Even though nerve fibers, nerve cells, and glial cells are often stained especially well, sometimes cells and fibers of cartilage, muscle, and connective tissue are adventitiously stained.

From the procedure described above it is obvious not only that the technique is difficult, but also that a great deal of time is required for its use. Unfortunately, aside from the tissue of the sympathetic nervous system, the retina is the most difficult to stain with chromium-silver. Therefore it is not the method of choice when beginning a reexamination of retinal structure. When impregnation does occur, however, pictures unequaled in beauty are produced. The structure of the Purkinje cells of the cerebellum or of the neuroglia cells ("Spinnenzellen") in the optic nerve is very instructive for learning the chromium-silver stain.[5, 6, 7] Here pictures may be obtained without great difficulty, and these make obvious how insufficiently and imprecisely such cells are represented with the earlier staining techniques, and also how clearly and extensively the morphology of nerve cells is shown with the Golgi method. Furthermore, one can see why this method has brought about such a great change in the conceptions of the anatomy and physiology of the nervous system. Figure 1 shows an example of a Purkinje cell in the cerebellum of the fifteen-day-old cat prepared by Cajal.[8] An abundance of

---

* In an article by Kallius ("Ein einfaches Verfahren, um Golgi'sche Präparate für die Dauer zu fixiern." *Anat. Heft*, 1893 [2].) the author attempts to avoid deterioration of the chromium-silver stain by treating the sections with a photographic developer, such as hydroquinone. In this way the metallic silver is precipitated out, and the preparations are thus made permanent.

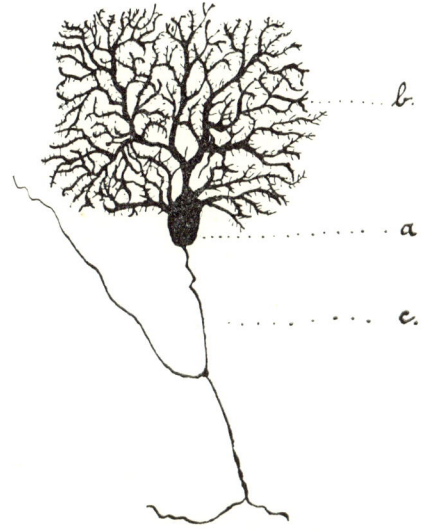

Figure 1. Purkinje cell from the cerebellum of a fifteen-day-old cat, from Cajal. *a* cell body; *b* protoplasmic ramification (dendrites), *c* nerve process.

ramifications of cell processes never before imagined can be seen.

The stained cells appear coffee-brown to deep black on a uniform dark yellow background. They contrast sharply from the background with all their very fine branches and look like a schematic textbook diagram. The staining is due to the conversion of potassium dichromate into silver dichromate by the action of the silver solution in the protoplasm of the nerves, thereby leaving the affected cells and their processes rather black. It was Golgi who first saw the numerous ramifications (dendrites and small terminal branches) of the protoplasmic processes of the nerves in such preparations. Soon after their origin the thickly gnarled protoplasmic processes divide dichotomously or in an antler-like fashion. The secondary and tertiary branches become smaller and smaller with continued divisions and finally terminate with countless tiny end-branches. A number of thickenings can usually be seen on the abundant and tangled protoplasmic processes. The branches often spread over an enormous area. It is to Golgi's credit that he demonstrated a fact which has proved to be a great step forward in the knowledge of the structure of the nervous system: namely, that *the terminal branches of all the protoplasmic processes of nerve cells end freely without fusing with one another or with neighboring cells.* Their endings appear either tapered or as a terminal knob. At the present time we can affirm the important fact that *nowhere in the nervous system does the formation of nets or anastomoses occur between the fine protoplasmic processes of nerve cells.* Gerlach still believes, however, that the network from which, for example, the lower root fibers arise, is made up of the confluence of protoplasmic ramifications of nerve cells.

The nerve-cylinder or axis-cylinder process may be easily distinguished from the protoplasmic processes in the chromium-silver preparation. It is much smoother and thinner than the protoplasmic process and follows a straight course. It looks rather like a "black thread on a bright background." In most cases only one axis cylinder is present, and it arises either directly from the cell body itself or from a protoplasmic trunk. The Golgi method stains only the axis cylinder and not the myelin sheath. Collateral branches often extend from the axis cylinder, as Golgi showed for the first time. This investigator distinguished two types of nerve cells on the basis of the course taken by the axis cylinders:

Type I. The nerve process retains its individuality and continues directly into a nerve fiber of the white substance (Deiters' cell type).

Type II. The nerve process divides shortly after its origin into a tree-like arborization (Golgi cell type, according to Waldeyer).

Golgi assumes that the Type II tree-like ramification enters into a common "nerve net": "This net is found throughout the gray matter of the spinal cord and is continuous with the fine nerve net of the medulla oblongata. It is present in a like manner in all layers of the gray matter of the brain."[9] Collaterals of Type I nerve processes also are present to enter this continuous net.

A further development must be recognized in Ramón y Cajal's

success with his careful investigations in disentangling this rich and complicated "network" by showing that the tree-like ramifying axis cylinders of the Type II cell and the collateral nerve fibers did not form a common network, but rather were found to be independent of the neighboring cells and to end with completely free terminal branches.

Thus, Cajal was successful in establishing a point which His had suggested in 1883 on the basis of developmental studies, and which Forel had predicted on the basis of theoretical considerations, i.e. that *there is total independence of the cells of the central nervous system from one another*. According to Cajal, the dense tangle of nerve fibers which can be seen so clearly in the gray matter does not form a network but rather a tight interlacing of nerve processes and extremely fine fibrils, all of which retain their autonomy and are simply pressed together and intertwined into a very compact feltwork.

The discovery of this fact, which has since been confirmed by many investigators, was a great step forward, especially for our understanding of physiological processes occurring in the central nervous system. Thus, a nerve stimulus is conducted from one cell to another, not through direct nervous continuity but rather by virtue of the fact that the processes of different nervous elements lie next to one another, or "come into contact with one another."

These are the principal areas in which we have made progress in our knowledge of the morphology of nerve cells with the new methods. I do not consider it superfluous to discuss briefly these modern advances in the field of neurology, since the new views concerning retinal structure are based on them. In reading this book, it can often be clearly recognized that the nerve cells of the retina are entirely similar to those of the central nervous system, i.e. *the retina is to be regarded as a peripherally-located nervous center*. It has been possible to establish and confirm all the laws of morphology and physiology of nerve cells in the retina. Indeed, we have an organ here which is quite well suited for learning about the structure of a nervous center, even more so than any other part of the central nervous system. Ramón y Cajal often comments on general neuroanatomy and presupposes some knowledge of the latest views. This brief introduction might therefore be welcomed by many readers. Cajal retains as a basic rule the doctrine of complete independence of nerve cells, all of whose terminal branches spread freely. *There are no nerve nets in vertebrates.* The importance which he assigns to this statement can be seen by the fact that he addressed the bulk of his studies on the retina to precisely this point.

* * *

The development of our knowledge of the structure of the retina is no less interesting. Here is a tiny organ (about 0.3 mm thick in man) which by its function and highly complex and marvelous structure has inspired many of our most eminent researchers to study it. We could review several hundred works on the retina, each being based on the preceding ones and advancing our knowledge only minimally by criticizing or confirming earlier studies, or simply being attempts with new methods. Taken together, however, they afford us a magnificent proof of how far human effort and conscientious research can, with time, solve even the most difficult problems. It is not my intention to go into the history of research on the retina. I should only like to draw attention to one thing which is now very appropriate for this chapter. This is the fact that it is easy to classify the history of research on the retina into different epochs, each of which is related to the discovery of certain methods. With the improvement of a certain technique a great and usually sudden advance can be noted, whereas the subsequent exhaustive studies must usually be content with meager though valuable new findings. It was perhaps S. T. Sömmering who conclusively summarized everything that could be seen macroscopically in the retina. Further advances were made when, at the end of the second decade of this century, the compound microscope was introduced into scientific research. The studies of this epoch made by many investigators, from Wharton Jones to Henle and Corti, were then greatly advanced, chiefly because the techniques for correctly hardening tissue and systematically making thin sections had been learned (1850-1860). The significant advances made with these improved techniques were associated mainly with the classical works of H. Müller and Max Schultze.

It would be unjust to underestimate the numerous subsequent works, as we are indebted to them for many beautiful isolated findings and for diligent use and improvement of the techniques. It is obvious, though, that since M. Schultze a really new period has not dawned, because in all of the textbooks discussing retinal structure, the classic schema of M. Schultze may still be found.

One needs only compare this schema with one made by Cajal himself or one based on Cajal's work (see Figs. 2 and 3) to become aware of the great advance suddenly brought about by the very new methods of Golgi and Ehrlich. Even if we do not assume that we have a complete knowledge of the visual process and the anatomical path taken by the light stimulus, at least we are much nearer to this goal than we could hope even a short time ago. Again we are indebted exclusively to a new method for such progress. This progress dates from the time we succeeded in finding a reagent which did not uniformly stain every nerve cell of an organ but stained only a few cells and all of their processes clearly so that connections could be seen among the dense chaos of fibers. These new methods (the Golgi chromium-osmium-silver stain and the Ehrlich methylene blue stain) depicted cells with a complexity and clarity, and an abundance and fineness of ramifications not even remotely expected. It is probably appropriate to conclude this short review with the words of Edinger.[10]

> The development of our knowledge of the retina is instructive not only for the history of possible errors along this long path, but also because it shows how each advance was based on an improvement in the method of investigation. Whenever an improvement was made, it was utilized in conscientious work and people followed the suggested path as long as there was something to be gained. Never, though, has the search for other paths ended. New paths were found and unsuspected things were discovered. One can thus easily recognize how very important the improvement of methods is for the acquisition of knowledge.

The new period was inaugurated in the year 1887 by a work of Tartuferi.[11] Using the Golgi method, Tartuferi obtained very noteworthy results which significantly expanded our knowledge at that time. Above all he was successful in demonstrating the true morphology of bipolar cells in the inner nuclear layer. He recognized that these cells have both an ascending and a descending process which ramified with one termination in the outer plexiform layer and the other in the inner plexiform layer. He believed that his chromium-silver preparations demonstrated a continuity between the bipolar cells and the cells in the inner and outer structures, i.e. an uninterrupted pathway of nervous conduction from the rods and cones through the retina up to the optic fibers.

Numerous industrious investigations by the Russian scholar Dogiel followed. He used the methylene blue stain on the retina for the first time and improved it so that it could also be employed on fresh retinal tissue. His works on the retina, done exclusively with the Ehrlich method, are listed below:

Dogiel, A.: Über das Verhalten der nervösen Elemente in der Retina der Ganoiden, Reptilien, Vögel, und Säugetiere. *Anat. Anz.*, 1888 (3), 133.

Dogiel, A.: Über die nervösen Elemente in der Netzhaut der Amphibien. *Anat. Anz.*, 1888 (3), 342.

Dogiel, A.: Über die nervösen Elemente in der Netzhaut des Menschen. Erste Mitteilung. *Arch. f. mikrosk. Anat.*, 1891 (38), 317.

Dogiel, A.: Über die nervösen Elemente in der Netzhaut des Menschen. Zweite Mitteilung. *Arch. f. mikrosk. Anat.*, 1892 (4), 29.

Dogiel, A.: Zur Frage über den Bau der Nervenzellen und über das Verhältniss ihres Achsencylinderfortsatzes zu den Protoplasmafortsätzen. *Arch. f. mikrosk. Anat.*, 1892 (41), 62.

Dogiel, A.: Neuroglia in der Retina des Menschen. *Arch. f. mikrosk. Anat.*, 1892 (41), 612.

Dogiel, A.: Zur Frage über des Verhalten der Nervenzellen zu einander. *Arch. f. Anat. u. Physiol., Anat. Abt.*, 1893, p. 429.

It was Dogiel's fortunate idea to conduct his first investigations on the fish retina, since its relatively simple relationships made the study of nerve arborizations much easier. In his first study with the methylene blue technique he was able to confirm many of the facts which had been recently found by Tartuferi using the chromium-silver technique, and he was soon able to make additional discoveries.

Dogiel grouped the nervous elements in the human retina into three ganglion layers:

A. The outer ganglion layer (outer reticular layer) containing,
   1. the subepithelial cells
   2. the stellate cells
   3. the bipolar nerve cells
B. The middle ganglion layer (inner reticular layer)
C. The inner ganglion layer (spongioblast layer)

The nerve fiber layer succeeded this, etc.

In the present book Cajal deals with this often when discussing and criticizing Dogiel, so that a complete account of the latter's findings is not necessary here. Dogiel is the most enthusiastic opponent of the contact theory.

The investigator who has succeeded in demonstrating the organization of the nervous elements of the retina most thoroughly and clearly is the Spanish scholar Ramón y Cajal. We are grateful to him for such valuable pioneering discoveries in the domain of the central nervous system. He has chiefly used the Golgi silver impregnation method, which he improved upon considerably, but also older staining methods, as well as the Ehrlich methylene blue method for control studies.

His works on the retina are listed below in chronological order:

> Ramón y Cajal, S.: Estructura de la retina de las aves. *Rev. trim. d. Histol. norm. etr.*, Numero 1 y 2. May, 1888.
>
> Ramón y Cajal, S.: Sur la morphologie et les connexions des éléments de la rétine des oiseaux. *Anat. Anz.*, 1889 (4), 111.
>
> Ramón y Cajal, S.: Pequeñas contribuciones al conocimiento del sistema nervioso. III. La retina de los batracios y reptilos. August, 1891.
>
> Ramón y Cajal, S.: Notas preventivas sobre la retina y gran simpático de las mamiferos. 1891.
>
> Ramón y Cajal, S.: La retina de los teleosteos y algunas observaciones sobre la de los vertebrados superiores. Madrid, 1892.
>
> Ramón y Cajal, S.: Nuevo concepto de la histología de los centros

nerviosos. *Rev. d. Cien. Med. d. Barcelona,* 1892 (18), No. 16, 20, 22 and 23.

Ramón y Cajal, S.: La rétine des vertébrés. *La Cellule,* 1892 (9), 121-246.

Ramón y Cajal, S.: Neue Darstellung vom histologischen Bau des Centralnervensystems. *Arch. f. Anat. u. Physiol., Anat. Abt.,* 1893. (A translation by Dr. H. Held of "Nuevo concepto de la histología. . . .")

Another study which has been concerned with the structure of the retina and which has employed both modern methods is that of Baquis.[13] This investigator made beautiful observations with the Golgi method on the retina of the pine marten, and they are conveyed quite clearly. He supports the notion of a continuous association of the nervous elements, i.e. the formation of nerve nets. Cajal cites his work critically in the present volume.

Yet another study is that of Fromaget.[14] This investigator attempted to circumvent the difficulty of obtaining good impregnation of nerve cells in the retina by macerating the tissue in Ranvier alcohol briefly before putting it into the Golgi solutions. The purpose of this was to facilitate the penetration of the stain into the porous tissue. It does not appear, however, that this procedure is worth repeating, since his figures in the *Archives of Ophthalmology* are very poor. Fromaget does not introduce anything new and only confirms the view of Cajal and others that the rods and cones are *not* connected continuously with the bipolar cells, nor are the latter connected continuously with the ganglion cells. Instead, the nervous conduction is interrupted several times, and transmission of the nervous impulse occurs from cell to cell by contact between ramifications of cell processes.

Another study concerned with neural structure is that of Retzius,[15] who presented a discussion of nerve endings in sense organs, including the retina, and suggested a schema for the organization of the nervous elements of the retina. He is an unequivocal adherent to Cajal's doctrine that every nerve cell is independent, that their processes end freely without forming any type of net, and that the association of cells occurs only by contact between their ramifications.

We have introduced a number of schemata of retinal structure, many of which have been suggested by Cajal's work. They probably best illustrate the great progress we have made recently. As far as I know, the schemata are the following:

> His, W.: Über den Aufbau unseres Nervensystems. *Berliner klin. Wochenschr.*, 1893 (30), 957-963, 996-1001.
> Kallius, E., cited in Merkel, F. and Zuckerkandl, E.: Sinnesorgane. *Ergebn. d. Anat. u. Entwicklungsgesch.*, 1892 (2), 251-260.
> Ramón y Cajal, S.: Neue Darstellung vom histologischen Bau des Centralnervensystems. *Arch. f. Anat. u. Physiol.*, Anat. Abt., 1893, p. 400.

It seems appropriate also to include Cajal's schema in this volume, presented here in Figures 2 and 3.

The most interesting aspect of these new findings is unquestionably the clarification of all the connections from the receptors to the optic fibers. (See Fig. 2.) Tartuferi essentially succeeded in seeing this by his recognition of the true nature of the bipolar cells.

The problem of the connection of the light-sensitive elements with nerve elements which conduct the light stimulus directly to the nervous centers was studied frequently and in detail by distinguished investigators, but until now, only in vain. Both so-called reticular layers had presented special difficulties for investigation, and for a long time no one was successful in tracing the processes of the bipolar cells out from the inner nuclear layer. Recently, however, Schwalbe[16] and Merkel[17] observed that the upper processes of the bipolar cells break up into very small fibers in the outer plexiform layer beneath the rods and cones. This finding has been well established with the new staining techniques, and in addition it has been shown—as was never expected—that the descending process makes direct contact via finger-like processes on the upper surface of the ganglion cells (Fig. 2, *r*). With this the problem is solved, and in the most simple manner the connections of the rods, bipolar cells, ganglion cells, and optic fibers are generally agreed on. The rod fibers end freely with a nodule, and this nodule is covered by terminal fibers of the upper processes of certain bipolar cells (Fig. 2, *x*); the terminal fibers are destined only for the rods and can be dis-

xxxii   The Structure of the Retina

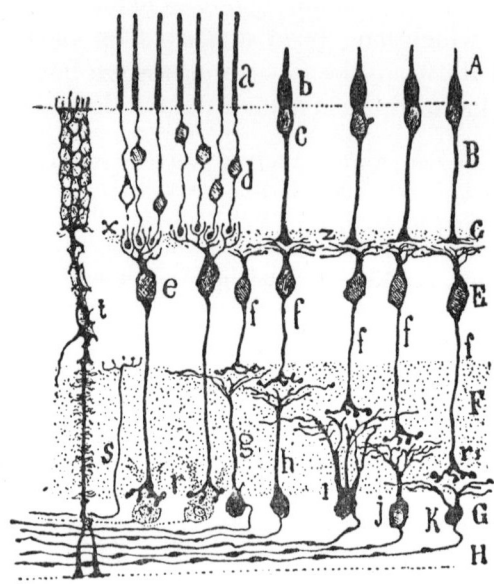

Figure 2. Schema for the structure of the retina, according to Cajal (representation of direct nervous transmission). A layer of the rods and cones; r lower arborization of the rod bipolar cells; r_1 lower arborization plexiform layer; E layer of the bipolar cells (inner nuclear layer); F inner plexiform layer; G ganglion cell layer; H optic nerve fiber layer; a rods; b cones; e bipolar cells destined for the rods; f bipolar cells destined for the cones; r lower arborization of the rod bipolar cells; r_1 lower arborization of the cone bipolar cell; g, h, i, j, k ganglion cells arborizing in different layers of the inner plexiform zone; z contact between the cones and the cone bipolar cells; t Müller or epithelial cells; s centrifugal nerve fiber; x contact between the rods and the rod bipolar cells; d cell bodies of the rods; c cell bodies of the cones.

tinguished from those belonging to bipolars destined only for the cones. These bipolar cells sit directly above a ganglion cell and surround it with finger-like branches. By means of such contact the ganglion cell conducts the impulse which it receives from the rods (Fig. 2, r).

The path through the cones is somewhat different. The cone fiber terminates with a wide base from which short basilar fibers extend. Contact is made with these fibrils by the ends of those bipolar cells destined for the cones. The lower process of these bipolar cells terminates at a different level in the inner plexiform layer with a terminal arborization.

These branches meet with the branches of certain ganglion cells which are directed upward (stratified cells). The branches interlace with one another, so that a small horizontal plexus is formed with neighboring cells which end at the same level. The five so-called sublayers, diagrammed in Figure 2 as successive levels of contact between two cells, arise in this way. In addition to the direct path of conduction, Cajal describes the new and highly interesting system of horizontal cells in the outer plexiform layer and the amacrine cells in the inner plexiform layer (cf. Fig. 3).

I have presented this brief discussion so that I can now examine the remaining controversial questions and newest criticisms of Cajal's work. Whereas in general the path which the stimulus takes from the rods and cones to the optic fibers is considered to be established, the form of the final cell terminations and the nature of the connections between the nervous elements

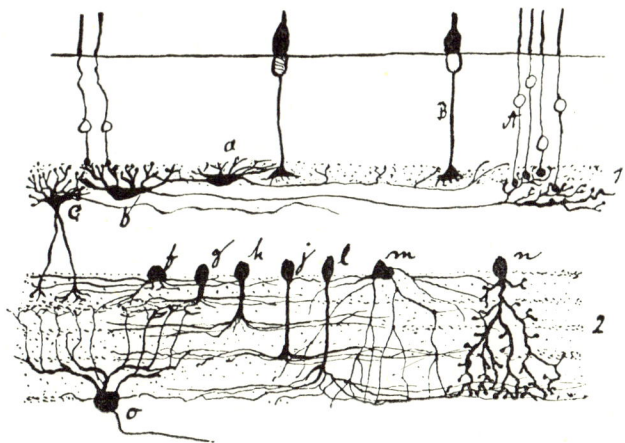

Figure 3. Schema for the structure of the retina according to Cajal (representation of indirect nervous transmission). A outer nuclei, or cell bodies of the rods; B cell bodies of the cones; a outer or small horizontal cells; b inner or large horizontal cells; c inner horizontal cell with a descending protoplasmic branch; e flattened arborization of one of these large cells; f, g, h, j, l spongioblasts, which arborize in different layers of the inner plexiform zone; m, n diffuse spongioblasts; o ganglion cells which arborize in the second layer; 1 outer plexiform layer; 2 inner plexiform layer.

is still subject to debate. Moreover, this is a question of great universal and principal importance, for anatomy as well as physiology and pathology of the entire nervous system. Should the old nerve net theory still remain valid, or should the new contact theory of Cajal be generally accepted today? When Cajal made his important discovery of the complete independence of each nerve cell and put forth the idea that an impulse is conducted from one cell to another only by the fact that the processes from both cells lie in close proximity to one another, the new doctrine was soon accepted by most important investigators and confirmed in subsequent studies by Kölliker, His, von Lenhossék, van Gehuchten, Retzius, Sala, and others. The nerve cells are individuals (Edinger) or neurons (Waldeyer) which are in no way connected with one another. The most vigorous opponent of this theory is Dogiel, who adheres strongly to the old nerve net theory on the basis of his preparations made with Ehrlich's technique. He has recently been successful in winning over some of our most eminent anatomists to his views. Thus, Waldeyer writes:

> I have at my disposal some of Dogiel's excellent preparations of the human retina, kindly sent to me by Dogiel himself. They convince me of the existence of net-like anastomoses, even though I had previously considered these to be very doubtful.[18]

Similarly Merkel declared:

> According to Retzius and Cajal, the ganglion cells ramify without forming an anastomosis with other cells. This view is directly contrary to Dogiel's. He says that the protoplasmic processes of all nerve cells of the retina join with one another and form nerve nets in both the inner and the outer ganglion layer. In order to make a judgment on this, preparations were made here in the institute according to Dogiel's specific procedures, and I assert that the stains which Dr. Kallius made prove that Dogiel's diagrams are completely correct. On the basis of these preparations it is not possible to believe that the anastomoses are illusions, and it is very easy to become convinced that in the inner ganglion layer at least an actual net of anastomoses does exist.[19]

The latest works of Cajal and most other investigators appear to oppose this view. Preparations made with the Ehrlich method may easily give rise to illusions. Because of the incomplete transparency of the tissue, fine fibers crossing over might be interpreted as anastomoses. If I compare the published figures of cells stained with methylene blue with those impregnated with chromium-silver, the latter show almost uniformly more abundant and extensive ramifications (dendrites). It is this condition which really supports Cajal's view of the independence of cells, for if there were continuity between cells, then they would have to be seen with the more adequate Golgi method. However, they are reported only by those who use the methylene blue technique.

From the above it can be seen that the question concerning the morphology and association of nerve cells, which is of great significance for the physiology of nervous conduction, has been studied mainly in the retina up to this time. Therefore, an interest in the structure of the retina is important for a number of scholars.

Merkel also denies the independence of the visual cells from the bipolar cells. In a preparation made by Dr. Kallius on the calf retina a fine fibril could be seen proceeding from the terminal swelling of a rod fiber and remaining in continuity with the extension of the outer processes of a bipolar cell. Of course this finding requires some consideration, but it was seen only in this one preparation. Cajal thinks that earlier investigators (e.g. Tartuferi, Baquis, Dogiel) who held that there were such processes on the ends of rods were simply reflecting the prejudices of a certain school. It was considered heretical to assume that cells as important as the visual cells should have no processes.

At the present time Merkel considers it to be unquestionably proven that there is merely contact between the processes of the ganglion cells and the descending fibers of the bipolar cells (inner nuclei).

There are still differences of interpretation regarding the nature of certain structures of the retina, i.e. whether they can be thought of as nervous elements or as structural substance. Cajal discusses this question often in the present volume. It is hoped that Weigert's neuroglia stain will further clarify this matter.

When we review the literature, we may be quite surprised at the advances which the new methods have brought about and also an especially great appreciation for Cajal's thorough investigations, which are presented here for the first time as an original work entirely in German. We are indebted to his studies on the retina for a number of new and important facts which were previously sought in vain. The path which a light stimulus takes through the retina is now largely clarified, and Cajal's findings with regard to this will never be subject to doubt. Opinions still differ somewhat on the manner in which the nerve cells are connected with one another, i.e. continuously or by contact. However, even Merkel, who still seems to be a bit skeptical of Cajal's views, states that today we need not be pessimistic about progress on the remaining controversial questions of retinal structure. We do not have to lay aside such questions, and we can expect to clarify them completely by proceeding along the present path.

REFERENCES

1. Kölliker, A.: Elemente des Nervensystems and centrale Nervensystems, *Handbuch der Gewebelehre des Menschen*, 6th ed. Leipzig, 1893, Vol. II, Part I, pp. 2-54, 55-89.
2. Golgi, C.: Sulla fina struttura dei Bulbi olfactorii. *Rev. sper. d. Fren.*, Reggio, 1875.
3. Golgi, C.: Sulla fina anatomia degli organi centrali del sistema nervioso. *Rev. sper. d. Freniat.*, 1882 (8), 165, 361. Also, 1883 (9), 1, 161, 385, and 1885 (11), 72, 193.
4. Ehrlich, P.: Über die Methyleneblaureaktion der lebenden Nervensubstanz. *Deutsch. med. Wochenschr.*, 1886 (12), 49-52.
5. Petrone, L.: Sur la structure des nerfs cérébro-rachidiens. *Intern. Monatsschr. f. Anat. u. Physiol.*, 1885 (5), 39-47.
6. Kallius, E.: Über Neurogliazellen in peripherischen Nerven. *Nachr. d. kgl. Gesellsch. d. Wissensch. u. d. Georg-August Univ. in Göttingen*, 1892, No. 14.
7. Michel: Über das Vorkommen von Neurogliazellen in dem Sehnerven, dem Chiasma, und dem Tractus optici. *Sitzungsber. d. phys-med Gesellsch. zu Würzburg*, 1893.
8. Ramón y Cajal, S.: Sur les fibres nerveuses de la conche granuleuse du cervelet et sur l'evolution des éléments cérébelleux. *Internat. Monatsschr. f. Anat. u. Physiol.*, 1890 (7), 12-31.
9. Golgi, C.: Sulla fina anatomia degli organi centralis del sistema nervioso. *Rev. sper. d. Freniat.*, 1882 (8).

10. Edinger, L.: Über die Entwickelung unserer Kenntnisse von der Netzhaut des Auges. Bericht der Senckenbergischen Naturforscher Gesellschaft. 1892, p. 166.
11. Tartuferi, F.: Sull'anatomia della retina. *Internat. Monatsschr. f. Anat. u. Physiol.*, 1887 (4), 421.
12. Tartuferi, F.: Sulla anatomia della retina. *Arch. per le scien. med.*, 1887 (11), 335-366.
13. Baquis, E.: Sulla retina della faina. *Anat. Anz.*, 1890 (5), 366-371.
14. Fromaget, C.: Contribution á l'étude de l'histologie de la rétine. *Arch. d'Ophthal.*, 1892 (12), 721-730.
15. Retzius, G.: Über die neuen Prinzipien in der Lehre von den Einrichtungen des sensiblen Nervensystems. *Biol. Untersuch., Neue Folge*, 1892 (4), 49-56.
16. Schwalbe, B.: Mikroskopische Anatomie des Sehnerven, der Netzhaut, und des Glaskörpers. In von Graefe, A. and Saemisch., T. *Handbuch der gesammten Augenheilkunde*, Leipzig, 1874, Vol. I, pp. 321-479.
17. Merkel, F.: Über die menschliche Retina. *Arch. f. Ophthal.*, 1876 (22), 1-25.
18. Waldeyer, W.: Referat über Ergebnisse der Anatomie und Entwicklungsgeschichte. *Berliner klin. Wochenschr.*, 1894 (10), 249-250.
19. Merkel, F., cited in Merkel, F. and Zuckerkandl, E.: Sinnesorgane. *Ergebn. d. Anat. u. Entwickelungsgesch.*, v892 (2), p. 253.

CONTENTS

	Page
Translators' Foreword to the English Edition—Sylvia A. Thorpe and Mitchell Glickstein	v
Translator's Foreword to the German Edition—Richard Greeff	xi
Introduction and Review of the Literature—Richard Greeff	xv

Chapter
- I. Introduction 3
- II. Investigative Methods 11
- III. The Retina of Teleost Fishes 17
- IV. The Retina of Batrachians (Frog) 39
- V. The Retina of Reptiles 60
- VI. The Retina of Birds 76
- VII. The Retina of Mammals 93
- VIII. The Fovea Centralis 133
- IX. The Development of Retinal Cells . . . 140
- X. General Conclusions 153

Publications of Santiago Ramón Y Cajal on the Visual System . 159
Legends for Plates 161
Plates 177
Name Index 191
Subject Index 193

The Structure of the Retina

Chapter I

INTRODUCTION

MY earlier research on the morphology and organization of nerve cells led me to the study of retinal structure. Several years ago I was able to discern new principles concerning the organization of nervous elements and the manner in which an impulse is transmitted from one cell to another in the spinal cord, cerebellum, and olfactory bulb. We now know that cells are not directly connected with one another by their processes, and therefore do not form a *net*. On the contrary, we know that the processes and branches of one cell lie against the tips or flat sides of a neighboring cell, and that effective transmission of nervous excitation from cell to cell occurs exclusively in this way. Cells enter into direct relation with one another only through intimate *contact* of their processes.

In my initial work on the bird retina,[1] I was able to confirm this law of cellular contact. At the same time, however, new and more difficult problems arose, which required continuous and exhaustive studies for their clarification. For this reason my investigations, which at first were restricted to birds, gradually were extended to include all five classes of vertebrates.

The retina has been the object of such a great deal of study that a complete bibliographic citation of all the relevant work would alone fill many pages.

The preference for the study of the retina shown by our most eminent anatomists and histologists can be understood easily if one recognizes the significance which the knowledge of reciprocal relationships between retinal elements has for the clarification of the visual mechanism and many related problems.

Interest in these studies is further heightened if the retina is regarded as a true nervous center, i.e. as a peripheral extension of the central nervous system, whose delicacy, transparency, and other structural characteristics make it especially suitable for histological analysis. In fact the cells and fibers of the nervous elements of the retina are essentially similar to those found in other centers; they are, however, more regularly arranged, so that different types of elements are distributed rather precisely in well separated layers. The following features are to be especially noted in the retina: (a) The protoplasmic processes extend over a small field. (b) The direction of the descending nervous process is known from the beginning and is always the same. (c) Layers are found which can be regarded *ex professo* as the site of intercellular connections (the inner and outer reticular, or plexiform, layers). Thus, unique and favorable circumstances are afforded here for clarifying the morphology and the interrelationships of nerve cells. For these reasons I thought that a study of the retina would shed light on the general problem of the connections and mechanism of action of ganglion cells. As I believe I have demonstrated previously,[2] such studies might even contribute to our knowledge of the direction of currents which travel through the protoplasmic extensions and the branches of nerve cells.

The history of research on retinal structure can be divided into two periods corresponding to the analytical methods which were used: (a) A period in which osmic acid or carmine staining were used, i.e. methods which were capable of staining only the nucleus and thick protoplasmic expansions of retinal cells. (b) A period in which chromium-silver and methylene blue were used, i.e. agents which could reveal clearly the protoplasmic processes and their finest nerve branches.

The first period consists mainly of the memorable work of H. Müller,[3] M. Schultze,[4] and the equally important work of Kölliker,[5] Hannover,[6] Krause,[7] W. Müller,[8] Schwalbe,[9] Boll,[10] Kühne,[11] Rivolta,[12] Golgi,[13] Ranvier,[14] Schiefferdecker,[15] Kuhnt,[16] and Borysiekiewicz.[17]

The findings of these enthusiastic workers are numerous and very important. The number of retinal layers as well as the morphological characteristics of nerve and epithelial cells were determined. With the help of osmic acid, a fixative introduced into microscopic technique by M. Schultze, the extremely interesting structure of the rods and cones has been studied in a precise way. Apparently there is a light-sensitive material in the outer segments of the rods (the "Photoaesthesin" of Boll and Kühne). Furthermore, the different types of cells scattered throughout the inner nuclear layer, e.g. the spongioblasts of Müller, the subreticular cells, have been distinguished from one another. Despite all these efforts two things remained unclarified: (a) the structure of the so-called molecular or reticular layers, and (b) the manner in which the fine processes of the retinal cells terminate. We also did not know the mode of connection between the endings of the visual cells and the cells of the inner nuclear layer or the outer reticular layer. The solution of these problems was left to the workers of the second historical period.

This second period, which might be called the epoch of methylene blue and chromium-silver, began in 1888 with the work of Tartuferi and Dogiel, and has been continued in my own work and that of E. Baquis. These investigators have given us a relatively exact knowledge of the termination of the nervous and protoplasmic processes of the retina because of the unique properties of the Ehrlich and Golgi staining techniques. Methylene blue and chromium-silver stain a given cell deeply out to its most peripheral and finest extensions while completely sparing neighboring cells.

Tartuferi,[18] who used the "rapid Golgi method," first showed that the ascending and descending processes of the bipolar cells terminated as a cluster ("en panache"). He also described the true morphology of several types of spongioblasts and subreticular cells and demonstrated the presence of axis cylinders in certain subreticular cells as well as giving details of the construction of the reticular layers.

Dogiel[19] took advantage of Ehrlich's methylene blue method, which he modified for use on the fresh retina. He was able not only to confirm Tartuferi's discoveries for almost all vertebrates, but also to make a number of equally interesting observations, such as the presence of Landolt clubs in the fish, reptile, and bird, and the occurrence of nerve cells with a descending process among the spongioblasts. Dogiel further demonstrated that the majority of the spongioblasts of Müller were specialized nervous elements which had no Deiters' process, and he established the existence of displaced bipolar cells* in the outer nuclear layer (subepithelial cells of Müller).

Despite this remarkable progress, certain questions still remained. How do the descending fibers of the rods and cones terminate? Do the lower terminal clusters of the bipolar cells form a "net" or a syncytium continuous with the protoplasmic branches of the ganglion cells? What types of spongioblasts are there, and what types of cells occur in the ganglion cell layer? Does the retina also contain centrifugal fibers? What role do the epithelial cells play,† and how are they arranged to form the framework of the retina?

These are the main questions which I have attempted to study since 1888, when Tartuferi's findings first appeared. At first my investigations dealt mainly with birds, where I could confirm many of the findings of Tartuferi and of Dogiel.[20] I then extended my observations to frogs, reptiles,[21] and mammals.[22] Most recently I have studied the teleost fish,[23] where the retinal structure may be especially suitable for helping to clarify certain questions which were obscure in the mammalian retina.

The most important results of my investigations are the following: (a) In the retina there are centrifugal fibers which terminate freely at the level of the spongioblasts where they break up into varicose branches. (b) The fibers of the rods and cones always end freely, as do the upper and lower terminal clusters of the bipolar cells. (c) There are collateral processes on the descending processes of the bipolar cells of birds, reptiles, and frogs.‡ (d) There are several morphologically distinct types of

---

* Cajal and Dogiel classify as displaced cells those cells which are found somewhere other than their usual location. For example, displaced bipolar cells are those cells whose cell body is almost in the ganglion cell layer rather than in the bipolar cell layer. These cells are identified as bipolar cells by their processes and connections. Compare also the interstitial cells. (Greeff's note)

† The Müller structural cells ("Stutzzellen") with their collaterals are to be understood here as the epithelial cells. (Greeff's note)

‡ Collateral fibers are classified as secondary branches of a nerve fiber which depart from the primary branch at right angles. The expression "collateral" simply refers to the fact that these branches are directed toward neighboring branches, and does not imply that they actually make connections with them. (Greeff's note)

ganglion cells and spongioblasts. (e) In nocturnal birds, mammals, and bony fishes, the fibers of the rods end freely with small swellings or knobs which have absolutely no "basilar fibers." (f) In mammals and teleost fish there are two types of bipolar cells: bipolar cells destined for the rods and bipolar cells destined for the cones. (g) At the level of the outer reticular layer there are several types of ascending and horizontal nerve fibers.*

Baquis' work on the retina of the marten[25] appeared after my first work on the retina. This author also used the Golgi method and confirmed most of the findings of Tartuferi and Dogiel. In addition, he described certain pyramidal cells which he considered to be new elements in the retina. I am inclined to think, however, that these cells are identical with those which Tartuferi had described as "large superficial cells." Baquis was fortunate enough to have stained these cells more completely than had Tartuferi and was therefore able to give a more detailed description of them. Quite recently Dogiel[26] stained these cells in the human retina with methylene blue and again pointed out the presence of an axis cylinder, which after a very long horizontal course descends and is continuous with an optic nerve fiber. He called these cells "large stellate cells" ("grosse sternförmige Zellen"). We will return to other facts which Dogiel reported when I describe the results of my own research on the mammalian retina.

The present work contains a résumé of all my earlier work on the retina which first appeared in Spanish and consequently was very little known by other workers. My monograph appeared in the French journal *La Cellule* in 1892, but a number of new facts and several corrections can be added to this; they have been incorporated into the present comprehensive German volume. Moreover, my investigations, which originally dealt only with the bird, have been extended to all five classes of verte-

---

* The ideas concerning the structure and physiology of the retina appear in recent works, where they are favorably reviewed. This is especially true of Retzius, van Gehuchten, and His.[24] The extensive investigations of Retzius are in good agreement with the opinions put forth here. (Greeff's note)

brates. Consequently, I am now in a position to expand the earlier results and to correct them partially.

The general conclusion which emerges from my work is the similarity of retinal structure in the vertebrates investigated. It can be asserted that the only anatomical variations which do occur are in the relative thickness of the individual layers of the retina, and in the shape and density of the rods and cones. It is mainly the rods, either because of their rather high density or because of the shape and extent of their lower terminations in the outer reticular layer which produce noteworthy differences. These differences are so characteristic that from this information alone one can determine the class of vertebrate. Conversely, apart from subtle variations, the cones present a nearly constant morphological picture.

It can be readily understood that every modification in the volume or form of the end-feet of the rods is correlated with differences in the form of the ascending clusters of the bipolar cells, and likewise of the subreticular cells (Dogiel's stellate cells). As we will see below, these differences are such that in some classes of vertebrates it is possible to differentiate nicely bipolar cells which connect with the rods from bipolar cells which connect with the cones. It is clear that such distinctions would be difficult or even impossible to establish in those animals in which the end-feet of the rods and cones have the same structure, as is the case in the retina of frogs and birds.

REFERENCES

1. Ramón y Cajal, S.: Morfologia y conexiones de los elementos de la retina de las aves. *Revista trim. de Histol. norm. y patol.* May, 1888.
   Ramón y Cajal, S.: Estructura de la retina de las aves. *Revista trim. de Histol. norm. y patol.* August, 1888.
2. Ramón y Cajal, S.: Significacion fisiológica de las expanciones protoplásmicas y nerviosas de las células de la sustancia gris. *Rev. de ciencias medicas.* 24 June, 1891.
3. Müller, H.: Anatomisch-histologische Untersuchungen über die Retina beim Menschen und Wirbeltieren. *Zeitschr. f. wissensch. Zool.*, 1857 (8), 1.
4. Schultze, M.: Untersuchungen über den feineren Bau der Retina. Bonn, 1872.
   Schultze, M.: Sehorgan. I. Die Retina. In Stricker, S. (Ed.): *Handbuch*

der Lehre von den Geweben des Menschen und der Tiere. Leipzig, 1872, Vol. 2, pp. 977-1031.

5. Kölliker, A.: *Handbuch der Gewebellehre des Menschen,* 1867.

    Kölliker, A.: Zur Anatomie und Physiologie der Retina. *Verh. der phys-med. Gesellsch. In Würzburg;* 1852 (3), 316-336.

6. Hannover, A.: Zur Anatomie und Physiologie der Retina. *Zeitschr. f. wissensch. Zool.,* 1854 (5), 17.

    Hannover, A.: *La rétine de l'homme et des vertébrés.* Paris, 1876.

7. Krause, W.: *Die Membrana finestrata der Retina.* Leipzig, 1868.

    Krause, W.: (Later works published on the vertebrate retina). *Intern. Monatsschr. f. Anat. u. Histol.,* 1886-1889.

8. Müller, W.: *Über die Stammesentwickelung des Sehorgans der Wirbeltiere.* Leipzig, 1874-1876.

9. Schwalbe, G.: Mikroskopische Anatomie des Sehnerven, der Netzhaut, und des Glaskörpers. In von Graefe, A., and Saemisch, T.: *Handbuch der gesammten Augenheilkunde.* Leipzig, 1874, Vol. 1, pp. 321-479.

    Schwalbe, G.: *Lehrbuch der Anatomie des Auges.* Erlangen, 1887.

10. Boll, F.: Zur Anatomie und Physiologie der Retina. *Arch. f. Anat. u. Physiol., Physiol. Abt.* 1887, pp. 4-36.

11. Kühne, W.: *Untersuchungen aus dem physiologischen Laboratorium zu Heidelberg,* 1878.

12. Rivolta, S.: Dello strato di cellule moltipolari che formano lo strato intergranuloso o intermedio nella retina del cavallo. *Giorn. d. anat. dis. et patolog. degli animali,* 1871 (3), 185-200.

13. Manfredi, and Golgi, C.: Annotazioni istologiche sulla retina del cavallo. *Giorn. d. Accad. d. med. d. Torino,* 1872 (12), 289-351.

14. Ranvier, L.: *Traité technique d'histologie.* Paris, 1875-1882, p. 952 ff.

15. Schiefferdecker, P.: Studien zur vergleichenden Histologie der Retina. *Arch. f. mikrosk. Anat.,* 1886 (28), 305-396.

16. Kuhnt, H.: Histologische Studien an der menschlichen Netzhaut. *Jenaische Zeitschr. f. Naturwissensch.,* 1890, 177.

17. Borysiekiewicz, M.: *Untersuchungen über den feineren Bau der Netzhaut.* Leipzig u. Wein, 1887.

18. Tartuferi, F.: Sull'anatomia della retina. *Intern. Monatsschr. f. Anat. u. Physiol.,* 1887 (4), 421-441.

19. Dogiel, A.: Über das Verhalten der nervösen Elemente in der Retina der Ganoiden, Reptilien, Vögel, und Säugetiere. *Anat. Anz.,* 1888 (3), 133-143.

    Dogiel, A.: Über die nervösen Elemente in der Netzhaut der Amphibien. *Anat. Anz.,* 1888 (3), 342-347.

    Dogiel, A.: Über die nervösen Elemente in der Retina des Menschen. *Arch. f. mikrosk. Anat.,* 1890, (38), 317-344.

20. Ramón y Cajal S.: Sur la morphologie et les connexions des éléments de la rétine des oiseaux. *Anat. Anz.,* 1889 (4), 111-121.

21. Ramón y Cajal, S.: Pequeñas contribuciones al conocimiento del sistema nervioso. II. Estructura de la retina de los batracios y reptiles. 20 August, 1891.
22. Ramón y Cajal, S.: Notas preventivas sobre la retina y gran simpático de los mamiferos. 10 December, 1891.
23. Ramón y Cajal, S.: La retina de los teléosteos y algunas observaciónes sobre la de los vertebrados superiores. *Trabajo leído ante la Sociedad española de Historia natural.* June 1, 1892. (Published in *Anal. d. la Soc. Esp. d. Hist. Nat.*, 1892 (2).
24. Retzius, G.: Biologische Untersuchungen. *Neue Folge*, 1892 (4).
    van Gehuchten, A.: Le système nerveux de l'homme Sierre, 1893.
    His, W.: Über den Aufbau unseres Nervensystems. *Verh. d. Gesellsch. deutsch. Naturforsch. u. Ärzte*, Erste Teil, Leipzig, 1893, pp. 39-67.
25. Baquis, E.: La retina della faina. *Anat. Anz.*, 1890 (5), 366-371.
26. Dogiel, A.: Über die nervösen Elemente in der Retina des Menschen. Erste Mitteilung. *Arch. f. mikrosk. Anat.*, 1890 (38), 317-344.

Chapter II

INVESTIGATIVE METHODS

IN my experiments on the retina I have used mainly the Golgi method (dichromate-osmium-silver stain) and the Ehrlich method (methylene blue stain). Recently I have also tried the Cox method[2] which Krause[1] recommends, although this gives results which are somewhat inconsistent. The results obtained with these three methods agree on those points which are most important for the structure of the retina. The method which best served me, however, was the "rapid" Golgi method, or impregnation with chromium-silver, which Tartuferi also had used. Individual cells are stained even to their finest and most distant ramifications, thereby making it possible to follow a single fine fibril. Most of the figures of the present volume show elements as they appeared to me after being stained black by chromium-silver impregnation.

In general the methylene blue stain was used only to check the results obtained with the Golgi method. The methylene blue stain is capable of giving equally brilliant and new results, as Dogiel demonstrated in this noteworthy work. For the most part, though, I have found it inferior to the Golgi method in clarity and completeness of staining. For example, methylene blue stains neither the fibers nor the lower swellings of the rods and cones. It also fails to stain the Müller fibers, centrifugal nerve processes, and some types of ganglion cells and spongioblasts. In addition, the retina is not completely transparent after it has been treated with ammonium picrate, or with a mixture of this reagent and osmic acid as recommended by Dogiel. Hence, it is usually impossible to trace the finest extensions of the nerve and protoplasmic processes, which accounts for the fact that in Dogiel's illustrations the retinal elements show minimal ramifications. Several mistakes have occurred in Dogiel's work because of this, e.g. the assumption of the existence of a continuous nerve net between the protoplasmic processes, an idea which is contrary to the investigations of His, Forel, Kölliker, von Lenhossék, van Gehuchten, Retzius, and myself.

In general I have followed Dogiel's instructions for the methylene blue stain. However, instead of removing the retina and placing it on a slide moistened with vitreous humor prior to staining, it was left in place (i.e. in the posterior half of the eye) and treated repeatedly for one to two hours with a solution of methylene blue. It goes without saying that the vitreous humor must be removed before staining and that during staining the tissue must remain in a moist chamber.

I fix the retina for two hours in ammonium picrate and then store it in a mixture of ammonium picrate and glycerin. The period of twenty-four hours in the fixative recommended by Dogiel does not seem advisable to me, since by that time the retina has swollen excessively, and the stain will fade to some degree.

Recently Apáthy[3] has suggested a syrupy mixture of gum arabic and sugar as a preservative. I have also tried this, with very satisfactory results.

An ordinary preparation which has been fixed in ammonium picrate can also be converted to a permanently fixed preparation by embedding in dry balsam or in Dammar resin dissolved in xylol. First the preparation is placed on a microscope slide which is kept warm in a steam bath. One or two drops of a concentrated clear gelatin solution (two parts gelatin, five parts water, two to three drops of saturated ammonium picrate) are then put on the slide. This solution must remain fluid for four or five minutes to allow penetration through the entire thickness of the tissue. The specimen is then covered with a cover slip which is pressed lightly in order to smooth wrinkles and retard subsequent shrinkage. Finally, after cooling, the cover slip is lifted. The preparation usually remains attached to the cover slip and is allowed to dry in the open air. Then it is placed on a slide which is coated with balsam or with Dammar resin dissolved in xylol. In this way the tissue will become quite transparent, and the staining of the cells will be very faithfully preserved.

The only drawback of this procedure is that the layers of the dried retina contract greatly, so that it is frequently difficult to determine at what level the impregnated elements lie. For this reason I use this method only for preparations in which a single layer of elements has been stained.

Moreover, one obtains better results with other tissues, e.g. the nerve endings in the cornea, the frog bladder, striated muscle fibers, etc.

The rapid Golgi method, which is so valuable for the clarity of its staining, is somewhat inconsistent in the small retinae of fish, reptiles, and frogs. In general it can be asserted that the smaller the retina, the more difficult it is to obtain good staining. For this reason I had to choose those animals in a given genus or family with the largest eyes. For example, excellent staining can almost always be obtained in *Lacerta viridis*, but only rarely in the smaller retina of *Lacerta agilis*.

Good staining, however, can be obtained in such small retinae as those of the frog, the adder, and *Lacerta agilis*, if the double impregnation method is used instead of the rapid Golgi method. I have suggested this method for other nerve centers, and it has been successfully employed by van Gehuchten and Retzius.

The procedure is as follows:
1. After removal of the vitreous humor the posterior half of the eye is immersed in a mixture of ordinary osmium dichromate (twenty parts of 3% potassium dichromate and five to six parts of 1% osmic acid solution).
2. When this solution has acted for twenty-four to forty-eight hours, the specimen is dried on blotting paper and then transferred to a 0.75%-1.00% silver nitrate solution for twenty-four hours.
3. Without prior rinsing, the tissue is returned to the same osmium dichromate solution, which must still contain some osmium. A few drops of osmium should be added if this is no longer the case. I have also used fresh solutions of osmium dichromate, but in this case the osmium content must be lower (20 gm of dichromate solution and 2-3 gm of the 1% osmium solution). A higher percentage of osmium does not disturb the stain, but it does

make the tissue too brittle. The tissue is left in the solution for twenty-four to thirty-six hours.
4. The tissue is placed in a new solution of 0.75-1.00% silver nitrate for at least one day.
5. The tissue is put into 40% alcohol for a few minutes and is then embedded superficially in paraffin and cut into thick sections. In order to facilitate the embedding, I put the retina on a paraffin block and work as fast as possible with a scalpel warmed over a flame. In this way the embedding medium does not penetrate the retina, thereby preventing desiccation. The sections are then washed for an hour in 40% alcohol and cleared in clove oil. The oil and paraffin are removed from the sections by washing the microscope slide with xylol. Finally, it is embedded in a solution of Dammar resin with xylol and is allowed to harden in a thin layer.

The greatest inconvenience which must be overcome before one can study the innermost layers of the retina is the presence of superficial deposits of chromium-silver crystals. I have been able to avoid these deposits by doing one of two things. Before placing the retina in the silver bath, it should be covered either with a very thin layer of celloidin (the celloidin should not be dry before the tissue is put into the silver solution), or with a fresh, pliant piece of animal tissue, such as peritoneum.

The simplest and most reliable way to produce the desired results is the following method, which is called the "rolling-up procedure" ("enroulement"; "Aufrollung"). After the vitreous humor has been removed, the retina is cut from around the papilla with a pair of scissors or a very sharp knife and then carefully separated from the choroid with a very fine brush. Then with the greatest possible care, one proceeds to roll up the retina such that the folds are touching one another, thus transforming this membrane into a solid cylindrical or spherical mass. In order to prevent the tissue from unrolling, it is rapidly coated superficially with celloidin (2%). After allowing a few seconds for the celloidin to harden, the tissue is placed immediately into the osmium dichromate solution. This rolled-up retina hardens as a compact mass and retains its cohesion as sections are cut. Sections may be made through the entire thickness of the block. On inspection of these sections under the microscope, one finds the retina cut in all directions, sometimes transversely, sometimes parallel to its plane, sometimes obliquely.

By use of the rolling-up procedure, one avoids entirely the formation of deposits on the surfaces of the retina. These deposits are found only in the most peripheral part of the block. Another advantage of this procedure is that since this tissue is very thick, one does not have to worry about excessive hardening. Whatever time is allowed in the hardening solution—one, two, or three days—it is still possible to find regions at some depth for which the duration of action is especially favorable. It is to this particular method that I owe the following: the discovery of fibers which branch in the outer reticular layer, the complete impregnation of the layer of optic nerve fibers and of those neuroglial elements in the area of the optic fibers of the retina, and finally, the opportunity to follow completely the protoplasmic branchings of the ganglion cells and the spongioblasts which often extend several tenths of a millimeter. Of course it is possible to combine this method with double-impregnation and even triple-impregnation discussed above.

This rolling-up procedure is especially suitable for the mammalian retina, but it can also be used with good results on all other vertebrate retinae. When the retina is medium-sized (rabbit, dog), it is possible to make *one* roll out of it, but in the large mammals (cow, sheep, horse), the retina must be divided into two or three pieces in order to avoid incomplete hardening of the inner zone.

Finally, for staining and hardening of the retina I have also used the following ordinary methods: carmine alum, acid fuchsin, hemotoxylin according to the Weigert-Pal method, etc. With these stains I was better able to determine the location of cells stained in my preparations with chromium-silver. Thin sections made with a retina treated by the Cox method offer the advantage that they can be treated subsequently with Grenarcher carmine without apparent alteration of the silver impregnation.

REFERENCES

1. Krause, W.: Demonstrationen von Präparaten der Retina von der Taube. *Sitz. d. anat. Gesellsch. zu München.* May, 1891.
2. Cox, W.: Imprägnation des centralen Nervensystems mit Quecksilbersalzen. *Arch. f. mikrosk. Anat.,* 1891 (37), 16-21.
3. Apáthy, St.: Erfahrungen in der Behandlung des Nervensystems für histologische Zwecke. Erste Mitteilung: Methylenblau. *Zeitsch. f. wissensch. Mikrosk.,* 1892 (9), 15-37.

Chapter III

THE RETINA OF TELEOST FISHES

THE most significant studies of the teleost retina have been done by M. Schultze,[1] W. Müller,[2] Reich,[3] Hannover,[4] Denissenko,[5] Retzius,[6] and W. Krause.[7] Krause in particular has very carefully investigated a large number of families from this order of fishes. Such investigations, which were done with the older methods, have demonstrated that the structure of the teleost retina is very similar to that of other vertebrates, aside from certain modifications in the subreticular cells and some peculiarities in the configuration of the rods (giant club-shaped rods, etc.).

I used the Golgi and Ehrlich methods in the hope of finding a simpler retina in these animals. Were this true, it would be of great help in interpreting the complex relations in the retinae of birds, reptiles, and mammals.

Because of the difficulty in obtaining the necessary material, the present study was limited to a small number of species of fish: among the Percidae, *Perca fluviatilis*, and *Box salpa*, and among the Cyprinidae, *Cyprinus carpio*, *Tinca vulgaris*, and *Barbus fluviatilis*.

We will follow the classical nomenclature of Schwalbe and Ranvier in differentiating the retinal layers, although I have introduced a few modifications which seem necessary for clarity and ease of exposition. Because our knowledge of the morphology and significance of certain retinal elements has changed vastly in the past few years, some earlier names are no longer useful, e.g. "reticular layers," "neurospongium," "molecular layer," "spongioblasts," "granular layers," etc. Such terms are related either to the gross structure or to incorrect notions about the structure or histogenesis of the retina.

The following nomenclature is a provisional one, based mainly on morphology. It has the advantage of not imposing a bias concerning the origin and function of retinal elements at the outset. Proceeding from distal to proximal are the following:

1. the epithelial or pigment layer
2. the visual cell layer (cones and rods)
3. the layer of the visual cell nuclei (outer nuclear layer)
4. the outer plexiform layer (inter-nuclear layer, outer molecular layer, or outer reticular layer of other workers)
5. the horizontal cell layer (stellate cells, concentric cells, basilar corpuscles of other authors)
6. the bipolar cell layer ("ganglion retinae")
7. the amacrine cell layer* (Müller's spongioblasts)
8. the inner plexiform layer (inner reticular or inner molecular layer, neurospongium, "Plexus cerebralis retinae")
9. the ganglion cell layer ("ganglion nervi optici")
10. the optic fiber layer

The Müller cells, or supporting tissue, and the neuroglial cells ("Spinnenzellen," "cellule en araignée") will be considered separately. The external and internal limiting membranes cannot be considered to be separate and independent layers, because they are only the borders of the Müller fibers, and hence are studied along with them.

VISUAL CELL LAYER

The rods and cones of the teleost fish are well known for their enormous length. With the exception of the ellipsoid body, they do not stain with methylene blue. As described by Dogiel, who worked with the retina of the ganoid fish, the ellipsoid bodies take on a dark stain. Chromium-silver, however, stains the visual cells very effectively, although the stain is restricted almost entirely to the inner segment of the rods and cones.

The inner segment of the rod is very long and fine; it resembles a nerve fiber in its delicacy and varicosity. Often a sizeable varicosity can be found near the level of the cone nuclei, i.e. close to the outer limiting membrane (Plate I, Fig. 1, *b*).

In contrast to the inner segment of the rod, the inner segment

---

* In order to avoid the unacceptable designation "spongioblast" or a long descriptive phrase, I use the term "amacrine cells" for Müller's spongioblasts (α without, μαχρος long, ινος fiber, or literally, without a long fiber or axon).

of the cone is very large and thick. At its innermost part, just outside the outer limiting membrane, there is an elliptical nucleus surrounded by a thin layer of protoplasm. The diameter of the cone increases just outside the nucleus and then progressively diminishes (Plate I, Fig. 1, *a*).

LAYER OF VISUAL CELL NUCLEI

All nuclei seen in this layer are rod nuclei. The cones contribute only their terminal fibers to this layer. The cell body of the rod is very small and thus like that of the mammal. It is composed almost entirely of an oval or elliptical nucleus which appears coffee-brown in a chromium-silver preparation. The fibers of the rods are very delicate, varicose, and gnarled. They terminate entirely freely at different levels in the outer portion of the outer plexiform layer as irregular or spherical swellings having no ramifications (Plate I, Fig. 1, *c*).

If a section stained with carmine is examined carefully, very pale granular areas which sometimes look like vacuoles can be found in the region of rod end-swellings. This pale zone contrasts sharply with the lower portion of the outer plexiform layer and may be called the layer of the rod spherules.

The cone fibers are much thicker and straighter than the rod fibers (Plate I, Fig. 1). Moreover, they terminate as a conical swelling deeper than the rods, as we know from the classical studies of M. Schultze. On the lower base of these terminations are very fine varicose processes which terminate freely at variable distances.

It should be noted that the base, or footpiece, of a cone lies much deeper in the outer plexiform layer than the terminal swelling or footpiece of a rod; the former usually extends to the lower boundary of this layer. An occasional rod spherule, however, may be seen at this level.

OUTER PLEXIFORM LAYER

This layer consists of a very complicated plexus of protoplasmic expansions and terminal arborizations of nerves. Two zones can be distinguished within this layer: (a) the deep zone, containing the cone pedicles, the upper processes of certain bipolar cells, and terminal ramifications of ascending nerve fibrils; (b) the superficial zone, containing the junction of most of the rod spherules, and the ascending processes of certain giant bipolar cells (bipolar cells associated with the rods). In addition, there are ramifications common to both zones. These include the numerous branches arising from the three rows of horizontal cells (subreticular or stellate cells of other investigators).

HORIZONTAL CELL LAYER

The very large cells of this layer are arranged in three layers which constitute most of the outer half of what other investigators have called the inner granular layer. These cells will be differentiated by the layer they occupy: *outer horizontal cells, middle horizontal cells,* and *inner horizontal cells.*

A. Outer Horizontal Cells

These cells (Plate I, Fig. 2, *a*) correspond to the membrana finestrata of W. Krause and to the intermediate concentric cells of Schiefferdecker. They are crowded together in a compact row directly below the outer plexiform layer. Despite many attempts, it was impossible to impregnate these elements with methylene blue; the Golgi method, however, proved successful in staining these cells. In such sections they appear as thick, black, four-sided or irregularly-shaped masses with short processes arising from their upper surface and extending into the outer plexiform layer, where they end with rounded terminal knobs. A long, fine branch which extends laterally from the cell body or from one of its peripheral processes can be regarded as an axis cylinder with a horizontal direction (Plate I, Fig. 2, *a*). The destination of this nerve process could not be determined in my investigations. If an analogy may be allowed, I would like to assume that this nerve process terminates freely in the outer plexiform layer with varicose branches. This is precisely what happens in these same cells in the birds, as we shall see later.

In this first layer no processes are sent out from the lower surface of the horizontal cells. It is always possible, however, to see a few branches extending laterally from the cell and ascending diagonally until they disappear in the outer plexiform layer. These appendages give the cells a stellate appearance when viewed in a horizontal section. They have been described by H. Müller, W. Krause, and Schiefferdecker.

The intimate contact between the edges and the processes of the outer horizontal cells makes it almost impossible to determine whether there are anastomoses between their protoplasmic processes. It is my opinion, however, that the net which Schiefferdecker and Krause describe (as the "membrana finestrata") simply demonstrates that it is impossible to distinguish the outer borders of the protoplasmic processes in horizontal sections which have been stained with the usual methods. The boundaries of the processes of these cells are very pale and undefined. They all extend along the same horizontal level and are tightly interwoven. It is interesting to recall that in other vertebrates it is easy to show a complete independence of these processes. Even in teleosts, there is no doubt that at least the ascending protoplasmic processes terminate freely with rounded knobs (Plate I, Fig. 2).

Between the edges of the outer horizontal cells there are spaces which allow the upper processes of the bipolar cells to pass through and also make room for the ascending processes of the intermediate horizontal cells from the second row. These spaces have previously been well-described by W. Krause, who thought they were gaps in a continuous granular membrane. Schwalbe[8] and Schiefferdecker have also seen and described them.

B. Intermediate Horizontal Cells

These cells, the second row of horizontal cells, lie in a virtually continuous layer just below the outer horizontal cells to which they are closely related morphologically. The cell body is flatter than the cells above them, and three, four, or more processes arise from the upper and lateral surfaces (Fig. 2, *b*). After these processes pass between the outer horizontal cells, they end in very short ascending branches which extend to the outermost part of the outer plexiform layer. Their tiny finger-like processes appear to be in contact with the rod spherules.

Just as in the first row of horizontal cells, there is often a long thin process which courses horizontally. It does not branch and looks exactly like a nerve process. I was not successful, however, in determining clearly how this process terminates.

The middle horizontal cells have already been well described and illustrated by W. Krause, Schwalbe, Reich, and Schiefferdecker, all of whose observations were made largely in the pike. According to Krause these cells are connected just like outer horizontal cells, so that their branches unite to form a continuous horizontal network. This is how the so-called "membrana perforata" of this investigator arises.

The perforations, which can be seen clearly in horizontal sections of the retina, correspond to the interspaces which allow the passage of the peripheral processes of the bipolar cells.

From what we have seen, we can conclude that the horizontal cells must in fact be thought of as true nerve cells. This fact has been well documented in higher vertebrates from the studies of Dogiel, Tartuferi, and myself. Satisfactory proof of this has not yet been demonstrated for the fish, and it is therefore understandable that Schiefferdecker included these cells in the supporting system of the retina, under the name of concentric middle and inner cells.

In ganoid fishes Dogiel[9] demonstrated the existence of roundish or ovoidal, cells lying above the outer plexiform layer, which he called "subepithelial cells." These cells evidently correspond to Krause's "Ersatzzellen" and have been found in the bony fish by Schiefferdecker, who considers them to comprise the outermost stratum of his structural system (his "outer concentric cells"). According to Dogiel's most recent publication,[10] these cells also appear in the human retina, and they are said to be displaced bipolar cells. Despite repeated attempts with both the Golgi and Ehrlich staining methods, I could not see these cells and therefore cannot affirm their existence in the teleost fish. In contrast, these cells are extensively developed and very characteristic in the frog and reptile retina.

C. Inner Horizontal Cells

These cells, the third row of horizontal cells, form thick elongated masses which lie directly above the bipolar cell layer.

They are spindle-shaped or semilunar with a superior concavity. (Plate I, Fig. 2, *e, g, f*). Usually the cell body sends out two thick processes which extend over a great length in two opposing horizontal directions. Near their origin, these processes are conical and show alternating thickenings and constrictions, but they gradually become finer and more delicate as the distance from the cell body increases. One of the processes looks like an axis cylinder. Over a long course it gradually approaches the outer plexiform layer, where it appears to terminate. The other process also takes a more or less horizontal course, occasionally bifurcates, and travels as far as the region of the outer plexiform layer, where it terminates in a manner which is still unclear. Because of its rough appearance and its size, this process seems to be a protoplasmic branch. Near its origin this protoplasmic branch often has an ovoidal thickening, which is very similar to the cell body. It is suggested that this could be a cell with two nuclei (Plate I, Fig. 2, *f*).

These fusiform cells are very abundant in the teleost fish. They are arranged in a layer which has a plexiform appearance. This layer is filled with pale vacuoles and has horizontal fibers running through it. This fibrillar appearance has not escaped the notice of earlier workers, having been mentioned by M. Schultze and Schwalbe. They accounted for it by assuming that there was a nervous plexus which lay over the spongioblasts and was continuous with the filaments which arose from the rods and the cones ("Plexus externe"). W. Krause, who was especially struck by the irregular vacuoles which interrupted the continuity of this region of the inner nuclear layer, called this portion of the retina "Stratum lacunosum." It is Schiefferdecker, though, who deserves credit for being the first to recognize these spindle-shaped cells and to give a morphological description of them. He considered them to be a type of supporting cell principally characterized by the lack of a nucleus ("kernlose koncentrische Zellen"). The fusiform cells in Schiefferdecker's figures correspond well with those I myself have stained with chromium-silver in Cyprinidae and Percidae. I would not, however, consider them to be supporting elements. As noted above, these cells do have an a axis cylinder; furthermore, they lack the morphological characteristics of neuroglial cells. I believe that for some reason Schiefferdecker was unable to stain the nucleus, since it would be quite remarkable to find nervous elements in the retina with no nucleus; all known nerve and neuroglial elements have a nucleus. Moreover, it is not difficult to see very nice nuclear staining with the Golgi method. With this stain the nucleus looks just like that of other cells (e.g. the bipolars), namely as a round and centrally-located body which has no black precipitate.

The three rows of horizontal cells just described are not peculiar to the fish. As W. Krause and Schiefferdecker have pointed out, they are present in all vertebrates with some degree of modification. Mammals, in this respect, are most similar to fish. Three rows of large horizontal cells are also seen in the retina of man, the dog, the calf, etc. The main difficulty arises in determining which cells in the mammalian retina correspond to the fusiform cells of the fish.

What function do these horizontal cells serve in the retina? In view of the present state of knowledge, any conclusions would be premature. If I may be permitted to conjecture, though, I suggest that these elements are for the mediation of lateral associative connections of the visual cells. This conclusion is based on the assumption that the axis cylinders of these cells terminate in free arborizations directly below the rod endfeet. (This type of termination has already been established in birds and mammals, as we shall see below.) For example, each horizontal cell of the first row would connect a small group of rods and cones with a similar group of rods and cones at a variable distance. The cells in the second and third layers would have an analogous function; since they have longer axis cylinders, they would connect two groups of rods and cones over a much greater distance.

BIPOLAR CELL LAYER

My investigations allowed me to establish a fact of some importance: there are two types of bipolar cells in the teleost retina. The first type is the *giant bipolar cell,* which is connected particularly with the rods, and the second type is the *small bi-*

polar cell, which has connections with the cones. Both types of cells stain with chromium-silver as well as with methylene blue (Plate I, Fig. 1).

A. Giant Bipolar Cells

These are very large fusiform cells; they are mixed with the smaller bipolar cells to form a thick and slightly irregular region above the "spongioblast layer" of other investigators. These cells have two processes, one of which ascends and the other descends.

The ascending process is quite thick and has an irregular appearance. It ascends virtually in a straight line to the outer plexiform layer, where it ramifies in a very rich and elegant tuft. The fibers branch repeatedly and eventually terminate as small knobs among the rod spherules (Fig. 1, *j*).

Since the terminal cluster of the ascending process is often very extensive, a single giant bipolar cell can make contact with a large number of rods, and thus integrate the impulses from these rods. Some bipolar cells form such a small upper terminal cluster, though, that they make contact with no more than four to nine rods. On the other hand, there are bipolar cells with ascending clusters that contact as many as twenty to twenty-five rods.

In comparison to the descending process of the small bipolar cells, the descending process of the giant bipolar cells is quite thick. It descends in a roughly straight line to the lower part of the inner plexiform layer, where it terminates in a conical footpiece which often has quite irregular, varicose, and thick lateral extensions (Plate I, Fig. 1, *f*). These footpieces are closely applied to the rather irregular upper surface of the ganglion cells or to the surface of the large ascending branches of the ganglion cells, thus forming an intimate articulation. This interesting association can be seen nicely in well-prepared sections.

The great majority of those giant bipolar cells which I could follow terminated directly over the ganglion cells. However I was often able to observe certain cells whose footpiece terminated in a more external layer (Plate I, Fig. 1, *i*).

It is very difficult to determine what type of ganglion cells receive the footpieces of the giant bipolar cells, although it appears to me that they are the giant or middle-sized type of ganglion cell (Fig. 1, *h*).

Those bipolar cells whose upper terminal clusters are small also have simpler and less extensive lower footpieces.

B. The Small Bipolar Cells

The cell body is small, fusiform, or oval, with a thin layer of protoplasm surrounding the nucleus. These cells also have two processes, an ascending and a descending one.

The ascending branch is very delicate and often bent. It courses between the horizontal cells above it and reaches the outer plexiform layer, where it breaks up into a flat bundle of elegant, fine fibrils. These fibrils are very long, and they follow a roughly straight course (Fig. 1, *e*). The terminal filaments form a horizontal plexus of modest thickness at the lower boundary of the outer plexiform layer, directly below the cone pedicles. These fibrils appear to be connected in a very special way with the cone feet.

It is very easy to differentiate the terminal clusters of these small bipolar cells, which are destined for the cones, from the terminal clusters of the giant bipolar cells, which are destined for the rods. They are distinguished by the fineness and great length of their fibrils, as well as by their perfectly horizontal course within the deepest portion of the outer plexiform layer.

The descending branch of the small bipolar cell is equally delicate and rather sinuous. It travels through the rows of amacrine cells, or the "spongioblasts" of other workers. At various levels of the inner plexiform layer it breaks up into a short, thick, and varicose terminal branch, which ends freely (Fig. 1, *g*).

Often the descending branch sends out a few small gnarled collateral branches that extend into one of the upper layers. This also occurs in the frog, reptile, and bird. On the basis of the relative expanse of the upper terminal cluster, it is possible to distinguish two types of these small bipolar cells: (a) those cells with clusters that are extensive enough to contact a great number (twenty to thirty) of cone feet, and (b) those cells with clusters that are so small they touch the terminals of no more than three or four cones.

It follows from the above that the specific excitation of the rods and cones becomes more or less concentrated as it passes through the bipolar cells, because of the fact that the lateral extent of the terminal cluster of the ascending process of a single bipolar cell allows it to receive and to transmit the excitation from a rather considerable number of rods and cones.

Small Stellate Cells

Within and above the spongioblast layer I have found cells whose morphological characteristics require us to regard them as a separate class of retinal elements (Plate I, Fig. 4, *a, b, d*).

These cells are very small (6μ-7μ diameter) and have stellate, triangular, or roundish cell bodies which send out a great number of processes. Their processes may be subdivided into ascending, descending, and horizontal types.

The ascending processes are very thin, delicate, and varicose, and thus appear similar to an axis cylinder. They ascend along a winding course in the spaces between the horizontal cells to the outer plexiform layer, where they form freely ending varicose horizontal arborizations. The final branches of the arborization lie in the lower part of the outer plexiform layer below the cone feet, where they mix with the plexus formed by the terminal clusters of the small bipolar cells.

Because of their relative thickness and regular contours, the descending processes—usually two, three, or four in number—appear to be protoplasmic branches. Initially they descend directly as far as the inner plexiform layer, which they traverse more or less diagonally, before terminating as varicose free endings. It is not infrequent to see these processes branch again within the same layer. Some of the secondary branches extend only a short distance before they terminate in the upper portion of the inner plexiform layer. Others have branches which are quite long and often reach the lower boundary of this layer (Plate I, Fig. 4, *h*).

The horizontal processes arise from a common stem, and because of their relative thickness, they also seem to be protoplasmic processes. They run horizontally at first, but soon ascend to the outer plexiform layer, where they terminate with lateral ramifications. Along their course they become progressively thinner and more varicose. As they travel above the amacrine cells, they also give off a few delicate ascending fibrils, which look like end-branches; that is to say, they break up into freely-ending terminations below the feet of the cones. Occasionally, rather than ascending, the end-branch doubles back and then descends to disappear in the inner plexiform layer.

Although we are not in a position to interpret the significance of these cells with certainty, I am inclined to believe that they are a variety of small bipolar cell destined for the cones. Nevertheless, these cells have a particular character which distinguishes them completely from all other retinal nerve cells: (a) The ascending processes appear very similar to a nerve fiber, whereas the descending processes are more like protoplasmic extensions. (b) Because of the irregular course of the descending branches, they do not resemble the footpieces of either the giant or the small bipolar cells.*

AMACRINE CELL LAYER, SPONGIOBLASTS OF MÜLLER

The same kind of spongioblasts which I described previously in the frog, reptile, bird, and mammal can be found in the teleost fish. As Dogiel has noted in the ganoid fish, these cells can be divided into two classes: the true *nerve cells*, and the *amacrine cells*, or cells with no axis cylinder (true spongioblasts).

A. Nerve Cells

According to Dogiel these cells have a miter-shaped cell body, horizontal protoplasmic processes, and give rise to a nerve process. The nerve process is said to penetrate the inner plexiform layer and eventually become a fiber of the optic nerve. Despite all my efforts, however, I did not succeed in staining these cells either in the Cyprinidae or in the Percidae. In my earlier studies I thought I saw such cells, but the staining was incomplete.

---

*I am now inclined to consider these elements as a variety of microglia, which have been thoroughly studied by the school of Río-Hortega. (1933 edition)

Further studies have forced me to conclude that the mitral cells which I did see were diffuse amacrine cells.

B. Amacrine Cells

These are a special type of nerve cell, as Dogiel has shown, since they lack an axis cylinder. Their branches can be regarded neither as functional expansions nor as protoplasmic processes. Amacrine cells can be compared with the granule cells of the olfactory bulb, since in both the two types of processes typical of ordinary nerve cells cannot be distinguished. They are also similar to the neuroblasts of His, i.e. primordial nerve cells which have been preserved in their embryonic state, somewhat like the type of ganglion cell found in invertebrates.

It would be possible to classify the amacrine cells by the shape and number of their processes. It seems more logical to me, however, to differentiate them by the type of termination and the location of their lower arborization in the inner plexiform layer. Using this classification they form two groups: 1. the diffuse amacrine cells, and 2. the stratified amacrine cells.* The former extend their flat branches within a definite sublayer of the inner plexiform layer, whereas the latter distribute terminal ramifica-

---

*Since the word newly created by Cajal is difficult to translate exactly into German, and also since experience has demonstrated to my colleagues and me that the anatomical representation of the relationships which have recently been discovered is not easy, the following brief commentary is given. The "cellules stratifées" of Cajal will be called "Schichtenzellen," or cells with branches that extend in a stratified manner. In this category Cajal included those cells whose processes projected over a rather wide area in the inner plexiform layer and broke up into a ramification at a different level. The so-called "étages d'arborisations," or levels of arborization, thus formed comprise certain layers or concentric plexuses, which we shall call the *sublayers* of the inner plexiform layer in order to distinguish them from the usual retinal layers. There are normally five such sublayers. There are (a) "células monoestratificadas," or single-layered cells whose processes extend into only one sublayer, (b) "células biestratificadas" and "células poliestratificadas," or multilayered cells whose processes extend into two or more sublayers. Stratified cells occur as (a) amacrine cells (spongioblasts) whose trunk descends and branches at a different level in the inner plexiform layer, and (b) ganglion cells whose trunk ascends and branches in the same level, so that both ramifications (that of the amacrine cell and that of the ganglion cell) come into contact with one another. In contrast to these stratified cells are the "células diffusas," or diffusely branching cells. (Greeff)

tions throughout almost the entire thickness of the inner plexiform layer.

1. Diffuse Amacrine Cells

There are two varieties of this cell: (a) Pyriform cells which are small and have a descending branch that rapidly divides into many twisted, varicose filaments. These filaments descend almost to the ganglion cell layer, and then terminate freely in a swelling (Plate I, Fig. 5, *M, L*). Sometimes these descending filaments will show considerable coarse varicosities in certain sublayers, especially in the third sublayer. The cell designated *N* (Plate I) in Figure 5 has its descending cluster directed diagonally and downward, and the majority of its filaments tend to accumulate in the fourth and fifth sublayers of the inner plexiform layer. (b) Ordinary multipolar cells with fine processes which are slightly-branched and course diagonally through the inner plexiform layer. They terminate at different levels, but especially in the fifth sublayer, which lies directly above the ganglion cells (Plate I, Fig. 2, *B*).

2. Stratified Amacrine Cells

Before beginning to describe these cells, we must examine certain structural details of the inner plexiform layer. All investigators have mentioned the existence of certain granular concentric stripes at various levels within the inner plexiform layer, but so far an interpretation of them has not been possible. Ranvier,[11] however, has suggested that these granular lines represent a cross section of different concentric plexuses, which are formed by the processes of spongioblasts and ganglion cells in the inner plexiform layer. But Dogiel deserves credit for having first demonstrated this to be the case, using the Ehrlich method, in four vertebrates: fish, frog, reptile, and bird. I have also confirmed this arrangement in birds by using the Golgi method.[12] Baquis[13] and Dogiel[14] later used the Golgi method to demonstrate it in mammals.

Although all recent investigators concerned with this matter agree on the existence of horizontal plexuses in the inner plexiform layer, they do not agree on the number of such plexuses.

Dogiel mentions three plexuses in his study on the bird retina: the first lies on the outer boundary of the inner plexiform layer; the second, in the upper third, and the last, near the lower boundary of this layer. In my first study on the retina (of the bird) I reported four such plexuses which were described under the name of *étages d'arborizations*. After some hesitation, though, I have subsequently become convinced that there are five plexuses, three of which lie within the inner plexiform layer and two—an inner one and a lower one—at the borders of this layer. It is possible, though, that there are even more plexuses, especially in the retinae of reptiles and birds, where the inner plexiform layer is especially thick and well developed. The number of plexuses appears to be related to the quantity and size of the bipolar cells: the smaller and more numerous the bipolar cells in a particular animal, usually the more plexuses there are. The five sublayers are difficult to demonstrate in the teleost fish and in mammals, because they lie so very close to one another, and also because the third plexus appears somewhat atrophied in the peripheral portions of the retina.

Every horizontal plexus of the inner plexiform layer appears to be formed by two strata of rather dense arborizations. The upper stratum is composed of branches of the stratified spongioblasts, while the lower stratum is composed of protoplasmic branches of the stratified ganglion cells. It seems likely that the irregular footpieces of the bipolar cells lie between these two strata, except for those which make contact with the upper surface of the ganglion cells, as described earlier. The boundaries of all the concentric layers are intimately connected with one another, either by Müller fibers or by numerous irregular and diverging fibers which arise from the nonstratified amacrine and ganglion cells.

The amacrine cells can be classified according to the level in the inner plexiform layer in which they arborize, thus giving us amacrine cells of the first, second, third, fourth, and fifth sublayers.

(a) *Amacrine cells of the first sublayer.* I have found two principal types: The first type includes very large cells which are hemispherical or semilunar; several thick diverging processes arise from their cell bodies, divide, and terminate exclusively in the external half of the first sublayer (Plate I, Fig. 5, A, B). The second type includes cuboidal or semilunar cells with many thin extensive processes which arise from the peripheral protoplasm and extend over a great area without dividing (Fig. 2, A).

(b) *Amacrine cells of the second sublayer.* There are also two varieties of these cells: The first type is pyriform cells which have a descending process that divides into twisted and varicose branches in the second sublayer (Plate I, Fig. 5, J). The second type is larger polygonal or pyriform cells which also have one descending trunk. This trunk forms a flat ramification with long, very fine, and virtually straight fibers at the boundary of the second sublayer (Plate I, Fig. 5, C). The fineness and delicacy of the contours of these fibers are reminiscent of the fine axis cylinders of the cerebellum (parallel fibers of the granule cells). These unique cells with stellate or radiating clusters can be found in all vertebrates.

(c) *Amacrine cells of the third sublayer.* Two main types can be recognized: one large, and the other small. The large cells are pyriform in shape (Plate I, Fig. 5, D). They have a thick descending trunk which breaks up into a flat arborization with relatively few, but thick, radiating branches. The small cells (Plate I, Fig. 5, E) are also pyriform, but they have a relatively slim descending trunk which forms an elegant stellate radiation exactly like the one described above (the second variety in the second sublayer) at the level of the third sublayer. The radiation is thus composed of very fine, long filaments which are independent of one another until they terminate freely.

(d) *Amacrine cells of the fourth sublayer.* There are also two types of these cells: giant cells with very large branches (Plate I, Fig. 5, H), and small cells with a slender trunk which divides into a number of straight, radiating, varicose fibers (Plate I, Fig. 5, O). The second type is sometimes as large as the first type (Plate I, Fig. 5, F).

(e) *Amacrine cells of the fifth sublayer.* I have recognized three types of cells in this layer, two of which correspond exactly to those described in the other layers. There is a giant type of cell with a few thick terminal branches (Plate I, Fig. 5, *I*), and a type of cell which is not as large, but has a very rich terminal ramification with numerous long, fine terminal branches (Plate I, Fig. 5, *G*). The third type of cell is usually multipolar (Plate I, Fig. 2, *B*) and sends out a fair number of branches to descend diagonally and terminate largely in the fifth sublayer, where they continue to divide and end freely. It is not infrequent that individual branches of these cells are given off in other sublayers.

Two-layered amacrine cells ("células biestratificadas"). It is not unusual to find a giant or rather large cell which is pyriform or semilunar in shape. In addition to their flat terminal ramifications destined for the third, fourth, or fifth sublayers, they also give off branches to the first sublayer (Plate I, Fig. 2, *C*). It often appears as though there are also processes from these cells which extend into the space between two retinal sublayers, thereby giving to the multistratified cells the appearance of diffusely branching cells.

INNER PLEXIFORM LAYER

This layer, as we have indicated, is formed mainly from the aggregation and interlacing of four types of terminal ramifications: (a) The protoplasmic ramifications of the ganglion cells, (b) the lower terminal clusters of the bipolar cells, (c) the terminal ramifications of the amacrine cells, (d) the lateral processes of the Müller fibers.

Cells of the Inner Plexiform Layer

If one looks at thin sections through the teleost retina stained with carmine or hemotoxylin, it is possible to see an occasional ovoidal or ellipsoidal nucleus surrounded by a triangular or fusiform body. Such cells have been observed previously in higher vertebrates by other investigators, especially Nagel,[15] H. Müller,[16] Ritter,[17] Golgi and Manfredi,[18] and Borysiekiewicz.[19] These workers do not agree on the nature of these cells: Some regard them as neuroglial elements, while others regard them as ganglion cells.

Fortunately, in sections impregnated with chromium-silver, it is possible to find some of these cells which have been well stained. Their features are shown in Plate I, Figure 2, *D*, where it can be seen that they resemble the spongioblasts. The cell body is triangular or fusiform and lies in one of the sublayers of the inner reticular or inner plexiform layer. Two, three, or more protoplasmic processes arise from the angles or protoplasmic poles of the cell body. These processes branch repeatedly and extend chiefly into the third and fifth sublayers. In the cell labelled *D* it can be observed that the final branches become more and more delicate and thin, resembling a nerve fiber. The terminal branches do not leave the inner plexiform layer, but terminate freely within it.

GANGLION CELL LAYER

Without exception the cells of this layer appear to be elements with long axis cylinders (the motor cells of Golgi). As other investigators have already mentioned, the axis cylinder always descends to the layer of the optic nerve fibers where it is continuous with one of these fibers. Throughout the long course of the axis cylinder neither collateral branches nor ascending free ramifications are observed. This fact is demonstrated especially well in horizontal sections stained with methylene blue.

Most of the protoplasmic processes ascend and terminate at various levels in the inner plexiform layer. There they terminate freely and are interwoven with the descending branches of the spongioblasts.

The ganglion cells can be divided into three groups by the form and location of their protoplasmic arborizations: A. single-layered cells ("células monoestratificadas"), i.e. those cells with terminal ramifications which extend within only one sublayer, B. multilayered cells ("células poliestratificadas"), i.e. cells which send out ramifying protoplasmic processes to several sublayers; C. unstratified or diffuse cells ("células diffusas," or "célules nonstratifées"), i.e. cells whose ascending ramification do not form a stratified plexus in any particular sublayer, but distributes diffusely through the entire thickness of the inner plexiform layer.

A. Single-layered Ganglion Cells

Corresponding to the five sublayers into which the ganglion cells extend their protoplasmic processes, it is possible to distinguish single-layered ganglion cells of the first sublayer, the second sublayer, etc.

1. Cells of the First Sublayer

I have found two cell types: (a) giant semilunar cells with two or three thick processes which arise from the upper surface, ascend, and ramify in the first sublayer (Plate I, Fig. 6, M); (b) middle-sized multipolar cells with rather slim ascending processes which form a very rich and varicose plexus in the first sublayer (Plate I, Fig. 6, G).

2. Cells of the Second Sublayer

The cells of this type which I have observed are shown in Plate I, Figure 6, I and L. They are small or medium-sized and send off one or more ascending branches which ramify repeatedly and end in the second sublayer, where they form a rather loose horizontal plexus. The final branches often look like small appendages or short collateral spines. These cells are not all of the same size; in fact, two types can be distinguished: small cells (Fig. 6, I) and middle-sized cells (Fig. 6, L). Perhaps there is also a giant type of cell with thick terminal ramifications similar to those I found in the bird, reptile, and mammal.

3. Cells of the Third Sublayer

These cells are pyriform and have only one ascending process. This process ascends to the third sublayer and breaks up into a plexus with fine, tiny varicose branches upon which collateral spines may be seen often (Plate I, Fig. 6, J, H). I have not yet observed a giant form of this cell.

4. Cells of the Fourth Sublayer

These elements are very abundant. Two types can be recognized: (a) a small pyriform cell whose ascending branch breaks up into a fine compact, and varicose ramification of rather restricted extent (Plate I, Fig. 6, *C*),* and (b) the middle-sized cell which has a multipolar cell body that is usually semilunar and has two or three ascending branches which form a horizontal plexus of thin, gnarled branches in the fourth sublayer (Plate I, Fig. 6, *F*).

5. *Cells of the Fifth Sublayer*

These cells are fusiform or stellate and are usually laterally elongated. Their rather thick branches—two, three, or four in number—extend almost horizontally and ramify in the lowermost part of the fifth sublayer (Plate I, Fig. 6, *B*).

B. Multilayered Ganglion Cells ("Células Poliestratificadas")

It seems that these cells occur least frequently in the retina. Judging from my own preparations, the following types of cells occur: (a) middle-sized multipolar cells whose ascending processes form two loose, varicose plexuses. One plexus lies in the second, the other in the fourth, sublayer (Plate I, Fig. 6, *E*); (b) small multipolar cells which give off delicate protoplasmic processes in the fourth and fifth sublayers (Plate I, Fig. 6, *D*).

C. Diffuse Ganglion Cells

One often finds multipolar cells whose protoplasmic processes give off terminal ramifications throughout virtually the entire thickness of the inner plexiform layer. Unlike most ganglion cells, they have no tendency to form a plexus at any particular sublayer (Plate I, Fig. 6, *A*).

Certain oval or fusiform cells with fairly large cell bodies that are oriented obliquely might also be included here. They are shown in Figure 2, *E*. Their protoplasmic processes appear to extend throughout most, if not all, of the inner plexiform layer. My observations on this particular group of cells are incomplete, however, since to date I have stained only a few of them.

---

* It is possible that these small cells are similar to the displaced amacrine cells which are so abundant in the bird and reptile. (1933 edition)

OPTIC FIBRE LAYER

As we know, the optic fibers in the retina spread radially and show numerous varicose swellings. In the teleost fish the optic fibers are arranged in thick bundles which follow a straight course. In preparations stained with methylene blue, one can easily observe that every fascicle is composed of one or two thick axis cylinders and a large number of finer fibrils, which are separated by a transparent mass. The Müller fibers travel between the fascicles, and at their entrance they conform to the arrangement of these bundles.

Most of the nerve fibers are continuous with processes of the ganglion cells. However, some of these appear to me to bend at a right or obtuse angle and reach the upper region of the inner plexiform layer. There, perhaps, they terminate in free ramifications in the vicinity of the amacrine cells. As yet I have not succeeded in definitely seeing the way in which they terminate, although this is very easy to demonstrate in the bird.

MÜLLER FIBERS, OR SUPPORTING CELLS OF THE RETINA

As may be seen from Figure 2, Plate VI, these cells are very much like those seen in the frog and the mammal. They differ only in their thickness and the great extent of their processes, which are given off at the level of the inner nuclear layer. Another distinguishing feature is the considerable volume of their nucleus. In their course, at the level corresponding to the amacrine cell layer, the Müller fibers send out many descending protoplasmic appendages which branch and terminate within the inner plexiform layer. In contrast, these small processes are not present in the outer plexiform layer.

REFERENCES

1. Schultze, M.: Zur Anatomie and Physiologie der Retina. *Arch. f. mikrosk. Anat.*, 1866 (2), 175-286.
2. Müller, W.: Über die Stammesentwicklung des Sehorgans der Wirbeltiere. *Beiträge zur Anat. u. Physiol.* Leipzig, 1894.
3. Reich: *Jahresbericht der Anat. u. Physiol.*, 1873 (3) and 1875 (5).
4. Hannover, A.: La rétine de l'homme et des vertébrés. Copenhagen, 1876.

5. Denissenko, G.: Über den Bau der äusseren Körnerschicht der Netzhaut bei den Wirbeltieren. *Arch. f. mikrosk. Anat*, 1881 (19), 395-441.
6. Retzius, G.: Biologische Untersuchungen. *Neue Folge*, 1881 (1) and 1882 (2).
7. Krause, W.: Die Retina. II. Die Retina der Fische. *Internat. Monatsschr. f. Histol. u. Anat.*, 1886 (3), 8-38 and 41-73. 1885 (5), 132-148. 1889 (6), 206-223 and 250-269.
8. Schwalbe, G.: Mikroskopische Anatomie des Sehnerven, der Netzhaut, und des Glaskörpers. In von Graefe, A. and Saemisch, T.: *Handbuch der gesammten Augenheilkunde*. Leipzig, 1874, Vol. 1, pp. 321-479.
9. Dogiel, A.: Die Retina der Ganoiden. *Arch. f. mikrosk. Anat.*, 1883 (22), 419-472.
10. Dogiel, A.: Über die nervösen Elemente in der Retina des Menschen. *Arch. f. mikrosk. Anat.*, 1891 (38), 317-344.
11. Ranvier, L.: *Traité technique d'histologie*. Paris, 1875-1882, p. 972.
12. Ramón y Cajal, S.: Sur la mophologie et les connexions des éléments de la rétine des oiseaux. *Anat. Anz.*, 1889 (4), 111.
13. Baquis, E.: La retina della faina. *Anat. Anz.*, 1890 (5), 366-371.
14. Dogiel, A.: Über die nervösen Elemente in der Retina des Menschen. *Arch. f. mikrosk. Anat.*, 1891 (38), 317-344.
15. Nagel, A.: Die fettige Degeneration der Netzhaut. *von Graefe's Arch. f. Ophthal.*, 1860 (6), 191-235.
16. Müller, H.: Anatomisch-physiologische Untersuchungen über die Retina des Menschen und der Wirbeltiere. *Zeitschr. f. wissensch. Zool.*, 1857 (8), 1.
17. Ritter, K.: Die Struktur der Retina, dargestellt nach Untersuchungen über das Walfischauge. Leipzig, 1864.
18. Manfredi, and Golgi, C.: Annotazioni istologishe sulla retina del cavallo. *Giorn. d. Accad. d. med. d. Torino*. 1872 (12), 289-351.
19. Borysiekiewicz, M.: Untersuchungen über den feineren Bau der Netzhaut. Leipzig u. Wein, 1887.

Chapter IV

THE RETINA OF BATRACHIANS (FROG)

FOR the most part, my observations have been made on the common frog *Rana temporaria* and also on the toad *Bufo vulgaris*. I have not been as successful in staining the retinae of the salamanders *Triton cristatus* and *Pleurodeles Waltli;* hence, the following description and figures are concerned exclusively with the frog retina.

VISUAL CELL LAYER

The visual cell layer is impregnated only rarely with chromium-silver and even when a few of these cells are stained, recognition and differentation of them is hindered by the pigment cells. To avoid this difficulty, several authors (Boll,[1] Angelucci,[2] Ewald and Kühne[3]) have recommended that the frog be kept in the dark for an hour prior to enucleation, in order to demonstrate the pigment migration in the retina caused by illumination of the eye. The retina is then removed in yellow or red light, rolled up according to the method discussed in the section on experimental methods, and immersed for twenty-four hours in the osmium dichromate mixture.

Under these conditions, the pigment is seen to have retracted toward the choroid, so that the rods and cones can be easily distinguished. A few of these visual cells are stained almost completely.

Cones

The cones have the familiar shape that has been described by other investigators. The inner segment is thick and cylindrical, whereas the outer segment is very short and remarkably thin. The outer segment ends with a slightly rounded tip.

Red, or Common, Rods

Usually only the inner segment is impregnated; it is perfectly cylindrical (Plate II, Fig. 5, *a*). In the beginning of the outer segment it is often possible to see black longitudinal stripes, corresponding to the superficial furrows described by other workers. Instead of these stripes, however, in some rods very fine, dark, transverse stripes separated by unstained bands can be seen. This finding supports the idea of a laminated structure of the outer segment, which has already been suggested by M. Schultze (Plate II, Fig. 5, b).

Green Rods

In addition to the red rods, I was occasionally successful in staining the green or club-shaped rods, which were discovered by Schwalbe,[4] and described fully by Hoffmann[5] and W. Krause.[6] In my own preparations I was able to distinguish two varieties: (a) rods whose inner segment is thin and very long (true club-shaped rods); in the outer nuclear layer they are continuous with a fiber which has a nucleus in the intermediate part of this layer (Plate II, Fig. 5, d); (b) rods whose inner segment is stouter but narrows noticeably at the point of junction with the outer segment. Each rod of this type has a nucleus located in the same place as the nucleus of the red rod, i.e. in direct contact with the outer limiting membrane (Plate II, Fig. 5, e).

LAYER OF THE VISUAL CELL NUCLEI

In this layer three types of elements can be distinguished: the nuclei of the rods, the nuclei of the cones, and the displaced bipolar cells (Ranvier's "Cellules basales"; Krause's "Ersatzzellen").

Nuclei and Fibers of the Rods

It is possible to differentiate the nucleus of the common rod from that of the club-shaped rod. The nuclei of the former are ovoidal and lie directly below the outer limiting membrane, as was mentioned above. Their descending fiber is very fine and often a bit wavy; it terminates with a conical thickening in the more external region of the outer plexiform layer (Plate II, Fig. 2, b and Fig. 5, f). A number of short, diverging processes arise from the flattened base of this swelling and proceed downward to end freely at the outer edge of the outer plexiform layer, which lies below.

As stated previously, the nuclei of the club-shaped rods may lie either directly below the outer limiting membrane (rods with a thick conical foot) or in the intermediate portion of the outer nuclear layer (Schwalbe's club-shaped rods). The descending fibers of the former terminate in the same manner as the descending fibers of the common rods (Plate II, Fig. 5, h). The descending fibers of the latter, however, are distinguished by the most remarkable circumstance of coursing obliquely and then terminating with a conical swelling which is oriented almost horizontally (Plate II, Fig. 5, g and Fig. 2, c, d). Terminal fibers arise from the base and sides of this swelling. Sometimes a true conical foot is absent. In this case, the descending fiber doubles back on itself and becomes progressively thinner until it terminates with multiple branches (Plate II, Fig. 2, c_2).

Most of the club-shaped rods which can be found in a well stained preparation are continuous with an oblique nucleus lying below, but I cannot yet be sure that *all* visual cells of this type behave in such a way. This doubt arises from the fact that the visual cells rarely stain completely: Most often if the rods are well stained, their nuclei remain unstained, and vice versa.

Nuclei and Fibers of the Cones

The description of the nucleus and the fiber of the cone given by previous authors can be verified with the aid of the chromium-silver stain (Plate II, Fig. 2, a and Fig. 5, i). The cone fiber becomes noticeably thicker in the vicinity of the outer plexiform layer where it ends, in a flat base with horizontal fibers. The rather large oval nucleus is located midway along the fiber's course.

Usually the smallness of the space in which the feet of the visual cells terminate, as well as the extremely complicated interweaving of the basilar processes, does not allow a precise determination of the plane in which the latter lie. However, under especially favorable circumstances, it can be established that each variety of visual cell—the cones, the common rods, and the club-shaped rods—extends its basilar processes into a different zone of the outer plexiform layer. After very careful observation, I was able to distinguish three successive visual plexuses: an outer, a middle, and an inner one.

The outer plexus occupies the most peripheral part of the outer plexiform layer. It is composed of fibrils derived from the feet of the common rods and from the uppermost clusters of certain bipolar cells. The middle plexus is formed by the interlacing of basilar cone fibrils with those fibers of the upper clusters of certain bipolar cells. The deep or inner plexus is comprised of the ascending extensions of the bipolars and the terminal filaments of the club-shaped rods, i.e. those rods with oblique nuclei.

Double Rods and Cones

I have not yet succeeded in staining the double cones ("cônes jumeaux"; "Zwillingszapfen"). It is probable, though, that the rather large nucleus of the cone shown in Plate II, Figure 3, *a* belongs under this category of visual cell.

In contrast, the double rods ("bâtonnets jumeaux"; "Zwillingsstäbchen") stain very nicely (Plate II, Fig. 3, *d*). Their outer segments, as well as their nuclei, are in intimate contact, although their fibers descend separately and terminate in the outer plexiform layer with conical swellings which are slightly separated from one another. It is significant that one of the swellings descends deeper than its companion and distributes its basilar filaments at a different level in the outer plexiform layer. This situation has also been seen very frequently in reptiles and birds (double cones).

Displaced Bipolar Cells

These cells (Krause's "Ersatzzellen," Ranvier's "Cellules basales," Schiefferdecker's outer concentric cells, and Dogiel's subepithelial cells) have been seen in many vertebrate species by W. Krause, Dogiel, Ranvier, Scheifferdecker, etc., but Dogiel is the only one who succeeded in defining their morphological characteristics. This scholar originally studied them in the ganoid fish,[7] and more recently he has described them in man.[8]

He first recognized them as true bipolar cells, but ones which were not in their usual location (i.e. the inner nuclear layer).

In the frog these elements are scarce and very small, as Schiefferdecker has noted. Their oval and pyriform cell body lies just next to the outer plexiform layer and has two processes: an ascending and a descending one. The ascending fiber forms a true Landolt club and terminates freely with a varicosity at the level of the outer limiting membrane. Sometimes this process is not present, or else it is not impregnated with chromium-silver. The descending process is noticeably thicker and, very near its origin, gives off a few ramifications which are destined for the outer plexiform layer (Plate II, Fig. 1, *b* and Fig. 2, *f*). The fiber then descends vertically through the underlying layers and ends completely freely within the inner plexiform layer with a very varicose, horizontal ramification. Occasionally, this process sends out a few short granular collateral branches to the more superficial sublayers of the inner plexiform layer.

OUTER PLEXIFORM LAYER

As discussed previously, this layer consists of three superimposed plexuses. The plexuses are made up of the basilar filaments (of the receptors) and the clusters of the bipolar cells, as well as the protoplasmic and nerve branches of the horizontal cells.

HORIZONTAL CELL LAYER

I have found only two types of horizontal cells in the frog. One type gives off long processes and lies in the outermost part of the outer plexiform layer; these are the outer horizontal cells. The other type is thicker and has shorter processes. These cells lie somewhat deeper and are called the inner horizontal cells.

Outer Horizontal Cells

These are the smaller horizontal cells, and they lie at the most superficial level (Plate II, Fig. 1, *e* and Fig. 3, *e*). The cell body, which is triangular or semilunar, sends out very long, thin, ramifying processes. Among these processes there is one which is very delicate and fine, and especially long. From time to time this process sends out short, fine ascending processes which terminate with a small swelling among the feet of the visual cells (Plate II, Fig. 3, f). Here we are probably dealing with a true axis cylinder, whose course is horizontal but whose free ending is difficult to locate because of its extensive course. In two favorable cases I successfully observed the terminations of these fibers; at such a termination there are two or three varicose ascending branches.

Inner Horizontal Cells

These cells are remarkably large and are also distinguished from the outer horizontal cells by the fact that most of their protoplasmic processes are much shorter (Plate II, Fig. 3, g). These processes are very numerous, and they ascend to the upper part of the outer plexiform layer where they end with a small varicose arborization among the feet of the visual cells.

From the side of the cell body a process with the characteristics of an axis cylinder arises (Plate II, Fig. 3, g). I do not know where this process ends, although in certain cases I was able to follow it for a considerable distance in the outer plexiform layer. Dogiel, who studied the frog retina with the methylene blue stain, found only one type of horizontal cell, which he called "stellate cells" ("sternförmige Zellen"). But I could not say from Dogiel's descriptions and drawings to which of my two classes of horizontal cells Dogiel's cells correspond. In any case, it is certain that Dogiel saw neither the horizontal axis cylinder of the cells, which I describe, nor the ascending terminal branches of the protoplasmic processes characteristic of the larger type of cell. On the contrary, Dogiel notes the existence of descending processes and protoplasmic anastomoses within the outer plexiform layer. I cannot confirm this finding. Perhaps Dogiel was looking at certain giant bipolar cells when he described his horizontal, or stellate, cells.

Both types of cells which I described, however, can be found mentioned in the work of other investigators, although under different names. Thus I believe that my outer horizontal cells definitely correspond to those cells whose anastomoses form the "Membrana fenestrata" of W. Krause, to the "Cellules basales interstitielles" found in the toad by Ranvier, and lastly, to those cells which Schiefferdecker called "middle concentric cells." Furthermore, my inner horizontal cells are the elements which W. Krause believes to compose the "Membrana perforata," the "Cellules basales internes" of Ranvier, and the inner concentric cells of Schiefferdecker. However, since these investigators worked with older and inadequate methods, I could not accept their views concerning the relationship and significance of the horizontal cells. I am relying on many observations on all five classes of vertebrates when I maintain that these cells are neural in nature and that they may be interpreted as true nerve cells with very short axis cylinders, since their functional process begins and ends within the retina itself.

BIPOLAR CELL LAYER

The bipolar cells were described well by Dogiel, although he assumes the existence of only a single type of such retinal cell. In my own Plate II, however, it is obvious that there are two types of bipolar cells (Figures 1, 2, and 3). They can be differentiated by their position and size of their cell body, as well as by the extent of the upper terminal cluster. The two types of bipolar cells are 1) large or outer bipolar cells, and 2) small or inner bipolar cells.

Large, or Outer, Bipolar Cells

I have already described these cells in the bird, in which they have almost the same form as in the frog. The cell body is mitral or oval, and it lies directly below the outer plexiform layer at almost the same height as the inner horizontal cells (Plate II, Fig. 3, *j* and Fig. 2, *h*). Horizontal processes extend from the upper surface of the cell body, branch repeatedly, and ultimately end freely in the middle of the outer plexiform layer. A descending trunk arises from the lower edge of the cell body. It traverses the underlying layers and breaks up into a flat, very varicose, and occasionally rather large arborization at the level of one of the inner plexiform sublayers. Not infrequently, this trunk gives off several flat collateral branches along its course through the superimposed plexuses.

Several varieties of these cells can be recognized on the basis of the extent and configuration of the upper and lower arborizations. Thus, in some cells the upper cluster is very extensive and flat (Plate II, Fig. 3, j), whereas in certain other cells the cluster appears greatly reduced. In addition, several of these terminal fibrils may ascend to penetrate as far as the layer of the end-feet of the common rods.

Does the first type of cluster connect with the cones, while the second type connects exclusively with the common rods? Even though my observations make such a relationship highly probable, I cannot categorically assert that it is true.

The large or outer bipolar cells appear to have no Landolt clubs; at least I have never been able to stain them.

Small, or Inner, Bipolar Cells

These elements are arranged in several layers and comprise the greater part of the so-called inner nuclear layer. Their cell body is almost one-third smaller than the cell body of outer bipolar cells; it is fusiform or elliptical in shape. The nucleus fills most of the cell body, which is visible when impregnated. The large nucleus is stained a coffee brown color with chromium-silver, but there is a delicate layer of protoplasm surrounding it which stains darker. Two processes extend from the two poles of the cell body: an ascending and a descending one.

The ascending process is thick and sometimes varicose and twisted, thereby adapting itself to the elements which lie above it. When it reaches the outer plexiform layer, it breaks up into a horizontal cluster with thin and relatively short fibrils. These fibrils terminate in either a blunt point or a small swelling (Plate II, Fig. 1, f). Some of these filaments ascend after taking a brief horizontal course.

Dogiel agrees with Tartuferi that the fibrils of the upper cluster of the bipolar cells anastomose with one another, thereby forming a continuous net beneath the feet of the visual cells; this is Dogiel's "subepithelial nerve net." But here, as in every other organ of the nervous system, I could never demonstrate a direct continuity between the extensions of different cells, even though I have used the Ehrlich method in my recent investigations. *Besides, little confidence should be placed in the net-shaped appearance of retinal sections stained with methylene blue.* Even in preparations which have been very intensely stained with this reagent, it is impossible to know precisely the site of termination of the fine filaments of the upper clusters of the bipolar cells. Under such circumstances there is nothing easier than to mistake the superposition of two lightly stained fibrils for an actual anastomosis. Therefore, when complex points concerning retinal structure are involved, the Golgi method should be used always as a control for the results obtained with the Ehrlich method. It is my own regular practice to do such. If both methods do not give the same results, then I favor that picture obtained with chromium-silver, since it has that property of staining even the most delicate ramifications of the cell with an intensity and completeness unknown to any other stain.

The Landolt club[9] arises from the central part of the ascending cluster or from one of its thick branches. It is an ascending fiber discovered by Landolt in the Triton and salamander, and whose continuity with the bipolar cells has been established by many investigators, particularly Hoffmann[10] and Ranvier.[11] Quite recently Dogiel has thoroughly studied the Landolt club in the frog, using the methylene blue stain. I can confirm the description given by this Russian scholar in all its aspects.

The Landolt fiber is usually somewhat thicker than most of the other fibers of the upper cluster, and it often appears to be the direct continuation of the ascending trunk. It has an arched course as it ascends through the outer nuclear layer, accommodating itself to the nuclei of the visual cells. It ends with a pointed or oval swelling either within or just beyond the outer limiting membrane. In addition to this terminal swelling, another swelling is often seen lying somewhat deeper (Plate II, Fig. 1, *f*, *c*). After its origin the Landolt fiber often changes direction in order to go around the end-feet of the visual cells, as shown in Plate II, Fig. 2, *g*.

The descending process of the bipolar cell travels through the inner nuclear layer. At varying levels within the inner plexiform layer, the descending process breaks up into a cluster whose fibers are quite varicose and roughly horizontal. These fibers terminate in a roundish or oval swelling (Plate II, Fig. 1 and Fig. 2). Just as in the large bipolar cells, the descending trunk often gives off flat collateral branches which are destined for the superimposed sublayers of the inner plexiform layer. With regard to this point, bipolar cells can be found whose descending fibers give rise to branches in three sublayers, though not always in the same three sublayers, as may be seen in Plate II, Figure 1 and Figure 2. Other cells can be seen in which the descending trunk gives off branches in two sublayers (Plate II, Fig. 1, *d* and Fig. 2, *k*). Finally, one can also frequently find cells whose trunk extends only to one sublayer, usually the fifth one, where it ramifies (Plate II, Fig. 1, *g*). Sometimes the terminal branches are so extensive that they fill two neighboring sublayers (Plate II, Fig. 2, *t*).*

AMACRINE CELL LAYER

We will classify the cells of this layer (Müller's spongioblasts) into two categories, just as we did in the teleost fish: A. the *nerve cells*, or Dogiel's cells, and B. the cells with no axis cylinder, or the true *amacrine cells*.

A. Nerve Cells

These are voluminous cells which are usually mitral-shaped. A number of horizontal protoplasmic branches arise from their lower surface and ramify in one or two of the outermost sublayers of the inner plexiform layer. The axis cylinder, which was discovered by Dogiel, often arises from a thick protoplasmic branch. After traversing the entire inner plexiform layer, it becomes a fiber which is a part of the layer of the optic nerve fibers (Plate II, Fig. 2, *s*). Judging from the rarity of occurrence of such cells in my own preparations, these cells must not be very numerous.

---

* As yet I have been unable to establish a definite relationship between the form and level of the upper cluster and that of the lower arborization. For example, I cannot say whether the bipolar cells which make special connections with the rods end in a specific sublayer of the inner nuclear layer. (1892 edition)

B. Amacrine Cells

According to the type of terminal ramification, we may distinguish diffuse amacrine cells and stratified amacrine cells.

1. Diffuse Amacrine Cells

These cells (Plate II, Fig. 2, *r* and Fig. 3, *O, J*) have small oval or plexiform cell bodies which usually lie in the upper portion of the inner nuclear layer. One or two descending processes arise from their lower surface or pole and divide several times. Ultimately they break up into a varicose, elegant, and very dense terminal ramification which occupies a large part of the thickness of the inner plexiform layer. It is possible to differentiate two varieties of cells on the basis of the extent and form of their terminal ramification: (a) elements whose terminal ramification is sparse and composed of fine, descending fibrils which branch minimally (Fig. 3, *J*), and (b) elements whose arborization is very varicose and quite dense (Plate II, Fig. 2, *r* and Fig. 3, *O*).

2. Stratified Amacrine Cells

These cells are classified quite naturally, according to the order in which they send their ramifications to the sublayers of the inner plexiform layer: single-layered cells ("células monoestratificadas") of the first sublayer, the second sublayer, etc.; and multilayered cells ("células poliestratificadas").

(a) *Cells of the first sublayer.* These are small rectangular or semilunar cells whose lower surface gives off very long processes. These processes radiate exclusively in the outermost part of the first sublayer (Plate II, Fig. 3, *A*). Two types of cells can be distinguished on the basis of the relative thickness of their branches: those with stout expansions, and those with fine ones.

(b) *Cells of the second sublayer.* Two varieties can be recognized. The first is monopolar cells (Plate II, Fig. 3, *C* and *E*) whose very short descending footpiece breaks up at the level of the second sublayer into an elegant star of very delicate and extensive horizontal filaments (more than 0.2 mm long). The second is cells which are also pyriform but somewhat smaller, and whose terminal cluster is composed of short, varicose, and very dense fibers (Plate II, Fig. 3, *D*).

(c) *Cells of the third sublayer.* There are also two types of cells in this sublayer. The first type is pyriform cells whose descending trunk reaches the third sublayer, where it breaks up into a flat and very extensive stellate arborization. The fibrils of this arborization are straight; they never divide and faithfully preserve their original level within the same plane. They terminate as very small swellings (Plate II, Fig. 3, *F*). The second type is cells of similar shape but whose terminal arborization is composed of very twisted, varicose, and thick fibers (Plate II, Fig. 3, *H*). Sometimes it is possible to find yet another variety of cell, which is characterized by its giant cell body and a lower arborization composed of thick, slightly twisted branches.

(d) *Cells of the fourth sublayer.* The same varieties occur in this sublayer as in previous sublayers. The first is pyriform cells which send out a very long stellate arborization to the fourth sublayer. I could follow individual fibrils for almost a millimeter (Plate II, Fig. 3, *N*). The second variety is cells of a similar shape but with a much smaller terminal ramification which is dense and quite varicose (Plate II, Fig. 3, *L*).

(e) *Cells of the fifth sublayer.* These are pyriform cells with a very long, straight trunk. They are characterized especially by the fact that their terminal arborization extends into the lower portion of the fifth sublayer, i.e. directly above the ganglion cell layer. Here one also sees both varieties which have been mentioned previously: cells with short and tortuous arborizations (Plate II, Fig. 3, *M*) and cells with extensive radiating arborizations.

3. Multilayered Amacrine Cells

I have occasionally found pyriform cells which give off two superimposed ramifications: one in the second, the other in the third sublayer.

Not infrequently, one finds cells which may appear similar to these cells (Plate II, Fig. 3, *G*). They have a polygonal body which send out a descending branch that ramifies repeatedly. In this way a plexus of very fine fibrils is formed in the fifth sublayer, and another but less rich plexus is formed in the second sublayer. A few branches of the arborization in the fifth sublayer ascend obliquely and join those of the second sublayer.

The description which I have given of the amacrine cells in the frog retina does not pretend to be complete. On the contrary, I believe that further investigations using impregnation with chromium-silver would allow the discovery of other varieties of spongioblasts, such as certain giant elements which I have often seen in the reptiles and birds.

Despite the gaps which are still present in this description, in comparison to Dogiel's,[12] it appears complete. If one carefully reads those few lines which Dogiel devoted to this topic, he becomes convinced that Dogiel probably saw certain pyriform spongioblasts whose descending trunks break up into a flattened arborization: from the point of view either of the sublayers of the inner plexiform layer to which their terminal clusters are sent, or the differences in the shape of their arborizations. Here is Dogiel's text:

> Regarding the second type of spongioblast, it is club-shaped and larger than the bipolar cells. These cells lie at the outer surface of the Neurospongium. One or more processes extend from the lower surface of these cells and divide at a particular depth within the Neurospongium. The branches then run parallel with the surface of the retina. I cannot yet say with certainty whether the fine varicose fibers anastomose with one another. The processes of these spongioblasts divide at a level different from that of the inner processes of the bipolar cells.

If we consult the figure accompanying Dogiel's text we can see the level of the layer in which the spongioblasts and the lower clusters of the bipolar cells lie. The former extend to the second sublayer, and the latter, to the fourth sublayer. This demonstrates that this scholar was not successful in staining with methylene blue either the spongioblasts of the other sublayers or the numerous bipolar cells whose lower clusters occupy levels other than the fourth sublayer.

GANGLION CELL LAYER

As in the teleost fish, I have found single-layered ("monoestratificadas"), multilayered ("poliestratificadas"), and diffuse ("diffusas") ganglion cells in the frog.

A. Single-layered Ganglion Cells

It is quite likely that the same five varieties which I described in the fish are present in the frog. (This number corresponds to the number of principal sublayers of the inner plexiform layer.) As yet, however, I have found only three varieties in the frog: those in the first, second, and fourth sublayers.*

1. Single-layered Cells of the Fourth Sublayer

These cells (Plate II, Fig. 4, c and Fig. 6, e), which are quite numerous, form a nearly continuous plexus at the level of the fourth sublayer, and stain very consistently. They are small, polygonal or pyriform, and they have one ascending trunk which initially divides into two or four branches. When these branches arrive in the designated sublayer, they split abruptly into a granular arborization which is neither very dense nor very extensive, so that it can be resolved with a very high power objective. In addition it must be examined *en face* so as to understand its structure, for a profile view reveals only a flat granular mass that is coffee-colored or sepia brown (Plate II, Fig. 4, c). The terminal branches of this arborization are extremely twisted; they also have collateral spines which end with a varicosity. I am of the opinion that there is an axis cylinder, simply because I believe that I have already demonstrated one in the bird. I have not yet been successful, though, in impregnating this axis cylinder in the frog retina.

2. Single-layered Cells of the Second Sublayer

I have found two types in this sublayer. The first type is a giant pyriform cell with a single ascending trunk, which upon

---

* These particular cells are probably displaced amacrine cells. They occur throughout all classes of vertebrates, with the exception of the primate. (1933 edition)

reaching the second sublayer, divides into two or more remarkably stout horizontal branches (Plate II, Fig. 4, *b*). Sometimes smaller cells of this same type can also be seen, as I have sketched in Plate II, Figure 4, *f*. The second type of cell consists of a giant pyriform or semilunar cell whose large trunk breaks up into a loose terminal ramification with thick, tortuous branches in the second sublayer. This terminal ramification radiates over a large extent of the retina (Plate II, Fig. 6, *a*).

3. *Single-layered Cells of the First Sublayer*

Judging from my preparations, these cells occur infrequently. I have noticed especially a giant variety with a semilunar cell body and two or three branches arising from its upper surface. These branches ascend obliquely to the outer boundary of the inner plexiform layer, where they form a very rich, horizontal plexus which is quite extensive (Plate II, Fig. 4, *d*).

B. Two-layered Cells

These cells appear to occur most frequently. Usually they participate in the formation of two, and less often, three horizontal plexuses. They can be divided into three groups.

1. *The Giant Type of Cell*

This group is composed of multipolar cells which have a very large semilunar cell body. Two or three very robust ascending branches arise from their upper surface and give off collateral branches in the form of a flat plexus as they pass through the fourth sublayer. The branches finally ascend to the second sublayer where they ramify repeatedly, thereby forming an even richer and more extensive horizontal plexus than the one in the fourth sublayer (Plate II, Fig. 6, c).

2. *The Middle-sized Type of Cell*

These cells (Plate II, Fig. 6, *g*) are also multipolar. They send out three or four processes which ascend obliquely to the level of the second sublayer. There they break up into a flat arborization with very fine complex fibers. At the level of the fourth sublayer these processes give off a great number of thick collateral branches which extend horizontally, thus forming a rather thick plexus. One always sees small ascending fibers which arise from the thick horizontal branches of the lower plexus to join and ramify amongst the branches of the upper plexus.

3. The Small Type of Cell

These are monopolar or multipolar cells whose ascending processes are of moderate thickness. They form a very delicate plexus in the second and fourth sublayers (Plate II, Fig. 6, *f*).

C. Multilayered Cells

These cells usually form three superimposed plexuses. Two main types can be found in the frog. The first type is a multipolar cell with a polygonal or oval shape. The ascending branches ramify successively to form plexuses in the fifth, fourth, and second sublayers (Plate II, Fig. 6, *d*). The second type of cell has several ascending processes which, during their course through the inner plexiform layer, form horizontal plexuses at the level of the fourth, third, and second sublayers (Plate II, Fig. 4, *a*). The plexus is composed of extremely delicate branches, reminiscent of the plexuses formed by certain multilayered cells in the reptile. (See Plate III, Fig. 5, *B*.)

D. Diffuse Nerve Cells

Certain multipolar cells (Plate II, Fig. 4, *e* and Fig. 6, *b*) are often noticed which are small or middle-sized and whose protoplasmic branches ramify and terminate throughout almost the entire thickness of the inner plexiform layer without being arranged in a flat plexus. It is possible to differentiate two varieties of these cells: One is small and has very fine, complicated protoplasmic ramifications (Plate II, Fig. 4, e). The other is larger and has a loose but more extensive ramification (Plate II, Fig. 6, *b*).

OPTIC NERVE LAYER

The optic nerve in the frog retina exhibits virtually the same characteristics as that of the teleost fish. The fibers arrange themselves in bundles which diverge from the optic disc. Here they no doubt form what Nicati[13] described as a true chiasma, i.e. the fibers at the periphery of the optic nerve are directed to the internal region of the retina, and vice versa. However, there are also optic nerve fibers which do not undergo a crossing, but proceed to the nearest part of the retina.

Most of the fibers of the optic nerve, upon reaching the ganglion cell layer, become axis cylinders of the ganglion cells. However, several ascending nerve fibers which are in continuity with the nerve process of Dogiel's spongioblasts can also be seen. Also, but more rarely, certain other fibers which are usually very fine and which seem to go to the inner plexiform layer can be seen. I would like to say a bit more about these fibers.

In my first work on the frog retina,[14] I described certain straight unbranched fibrils which took their origin at some points near the lower boundary of the inner plexiform layer. They radiated out in all directions and participated in the formation of a horizontal plexus at this level. I was of the opinion that these fibers could be considered as the direct continuation of some of the fibers of the optic nerve layer, because I never saw a continuity between such fibers and the clusters of the amacrine cells or with the clusters of the ganglion cells. The characteristics of the fibers themselves argued in favor of this interpretation. They had all the properties of axis cylinders: They were extremely long (often exceeding 1 mm); they were extraordinarily fine, and they had neither ramifications nor very sharp contours. Since I have never succeeded in demonstrating *de visu* the connection of such fibers with optic fibers, and since I later found certain types of spongioblasts and ganglion cells whose terminal fibrils are delicate, straight, and very long, I must modify my earlier opinion regarding the nature of these fibrils. In the teleost fish, the reptile, and the mammal, there are quadrilateral or semilunar ganglion cells which give off a large number of fine, diverging fibrils in the inner plexiform layer. These fibrils extend horizontally through almost the entire thickness of this layer, and tend to aggregate at the level of the horizontal plexuses. It would be quite remarkable if these elements did not exist in the batrachian retina. I would therefore like to assume that they are present in the frog. With this assumption it is then possible to clarify the tiny radiating fibers which are encountered so often in the "double impregnation" procedure, which I discussed earlier. However, the reason that the cells of origin of these fibers do not stain is not known (Plate II, Fig. 4, g). From Figure 4, g it is evident that the richness of the upper cluster of these elements far surpasses anything else we know in this respect. Their fibrils ascend obliquely through the different sublayers of the inner plexiform layer, and aggregate preferentially at the level of one of these sublayers. They attain an enormous length without ever dividing, and they appear to end completely freely with a small terminal swelling.*

It is furthermore quite possible that certain radiations of fine horizontal fibrils, which extend from the upper border of the inner plexiform layer and occupy a great portion of this layer, arise from certain special spongioblasts which are extremely difficult to stain in the frog (Plate II, Fig. 4, h). In fact these elements can be seen in the fish (Plate I, Fig. 2, A) and in the mammal (Plate V, Fig. 8, A).

Fibers Which End in the Outer Plexiform Layer

In a few preparations made with the double impregnation method, I was able to establish the presence of very fine fibrils which extended from the lower part of the inner nuclear layer or from the outermost region of the inner plexiform layer. After a more or less tortuous ascending path, these fibrils reach the lower region of the outer plexiform layer, where they form a very varicose horizontal ramification that ends quite freely (Plate II, Fig. 3, i).

In one case I saw that several of these ascending fibrils arose from a small trunk which seemed to be a protoplasmic branch (Plate II, Fig. 3, h), but in any case, it very probably originated from an unstained cell lying at the amacrine cell level. The similarity of these fibrils to those which arise from certain specialized cell bodies in the teleosts (Plate I, Fig. 4) makes it very rea-

---

* The origin of these thin radial fibers constitute a total enigma in the batrachian retina. This must be clarified in further research. (1933 edition)

sonable to suppose that these same cell bodies are present in the frog. In the frog, however, it is very difficult, if not impossible, to stain them with our present procedures. I believe that repeated attempts at staining with slight modifications in the method should make it possible to establish the presence of these cells. I do not know the origin of the ascending independent fibrils which emerge from the inner plexiform layer (Plate II, Fig. 3, i and Fig. 1, h). However, it is possible that they are the same type as those just described, and that they arise from a descending trunk of a special cell body, of whose existence in the frog we already speculated.*

Optic Fibers Which Penetrate the Inner Plexiform Layer

Very rarely it is possible to find fibers of the optic nerve layer which, after passing between the ganglion cells, penetrate the inner plexiform layer in an oblique direction. They travel horizontally through this layer over a great distance (Plate II, Fig. 6, h). I do not know where these fibrils terminate.

Until now it has not been possible for me to find centrifugal fibers in frogs which ramify at the level of the amacrine cells, as I described in birds and mammals. Of course this does not prove that such fibers do not exist in the batrachian retina but only that in some animals they have a very weak affinity for chromium-silver.

NEUROGLIAL CELLS

Spider Cells ("Cellules en Araignée)

I have never observed these cells in the optic nerve fiber layer of the frog, although they are very abundant in birds and mammals. On the other hand, they can be seen very nicely between the nerve bundles which form the optic nerve. They are very large lamellated cells with very long ramifying processes which arise from their notched surfaces as flat branches. Chromium-silver stains them a coffee-brown color.

---

* They might also represent the peripheral course of certain centrifugal nerve fibers which arise from the optic nerve fiber layer and arborize in the outer plexiform layer. (1892 edition)

Epithelial Cells or Müller Fibers

These elements stain very easily, and in a transverse section through the retina, one can see all the details described by other histologists, particularly Schwalbe and Ranvier. Figure 1 of Plate VI gives a good view of the appearance of the Müller fibers. These cells send out lamellated extensions within the outer and inner nuclear layers and also at the level of the ganglion cells. They constitute a system of cavities, closed off in the horizontal sense, which serve to support and isolate the individual nerve cells. At the level of the amacrine cells there is often a number of descending processes proceeding from the Müller fibers. They descend a certain distance through the inner plexiform layer along with the descending trunks of the amacrine cells (Plate VI, Fig. 1, d).

Usually there are no collateral branches in the outer plexiform layer; in contrast, they are quite numerous at the level of the inner plexiform layer. They have small spines, sometimes branched and sometimes undivided, which because of their horizontal direction apparently serve to support and isolate the horizontal plexuses of the inner plexiform layer (Plate VI, Fig. 1, e).

When neighboring cells have been stained it is possible to see that their processes are separated to some degree at the level of the inner plexiform layer. Furthermore, the collateral spines which arise from these processes are in contact with one another at their sides and tips. The quadrilateral or irregular space thus formed probably serves to enclose the nerve fibers (the plexuses of the individual sublayers). From this arrangement it follows that connections mediated by a plexus are facilitated only within a single level of ramification (i.e. in a single sublayer) but that connections between subjacent sublayers of nerve fibers are very difficult, or even impossible.

REFERENCES

1. Boll, F.: Zur Anatomie und Physiologie der Retina. *Arch. f. Physiol., Physiol. Abt.*, 1877, pp. 4-36.
2. Angelucci, A.: Histologische Untersuchungen über das retinale Pig-

mentepithel der Wirbeltiere. *Arch. f. Anat. u. Physiol., Physiol. Abt.*, 1878, pp. 353-386.
3. Ewald, A., and Kühne, W.: Untersuchungen über den Sehpurpur. *Untersuch. des. physiol. Instituts der Universität Heidelberg*, 1878 (1), 37-455, (p. 421).
4. Schwalbe, G.: Mikroskopische Anatomie des Sehnerven, der Netzhaut, und des Glaskörpers. In von Graefe, A., and Saemisch, T.: *Handbuch der gesammten Augenheilkunde*. Leipzig, 1874, Vol. I, pp. 321-479.
5. Hoffmann, C.: Zur Anatomie der Retina. II. Über den Bau der Retina bei den Beuteltieren. *Neiderl. Arch. f. Zool.*, 1876 (3) 1.
6. Krause, W.: III. Die Retina der Amphibien. *Intern. Monatsschr. f. Anatom. u. Physiol.*, 1892 (9), 151-236.
7. Dogiel, A.: Über das Verhalten der nervösen Elemente in der Retina der Ganoiden, Reptilien, Vögel, and Säugetiere. *Anat. Anz.*, 1888 (3), 133-143.
8. Dogiel, A.: Über die nervösen Elemente in der Retina des Menschen. *Arch. f. mikrosk. Anat.*, 1890 (38), 317-344.
9. Landolt, E.: Beiträge zur Anatomie der Retina vom Frosch, Salamander, und Triton. *Arch. f. mikrosk. Anat.*, 1871 (7), 81-98.
10. Hoffmann, C.: Zur Anatomie der Retina. I. Über den Bau der Retina bei Amphibien und Reptilien. *Niederl. Arch. f. Zool.*, 1876 (3), 1.
11. Ranvier, L.: *Traité technique d'histologie*. Paris, 1875-1882.
12. Dogiel, A.: Über die nervösen Elemente in der Netzhaut der Amphibien und Vögel. *Anat. Anz.*, 1888 (3), 342-347.
13. Nicati, W.: Reserches sur le mode de distribution des fibres nerveuses dans les nerfs optiques et dans la rétine. *Arch. d. physiol.*, 1875 (2), Series II, 521-529.
14. Raymón y Cajal, S.: Pequeñas communicaciones al conocimiento del sistema nervioso. III. La retina de los batracios y reptiles. 20 August, 1891.

Chapter V

THE RETINA OF REPTILES

MY research has been concerned mainly with the retina of the green lizard, *Lacerta viridis*. I have obtained the best preparations with this retina, probably because of its relative thickness. I have also been successful with staining the retina of *Lacerta muralis* and *Emys europaea*, but not as frequently as with *Lacerta viridis*. Quite recently I have had the opportunity to study the very interesting retina of the chameleon, *Chameleon vulgaris*.

ROD AND CONE LAYER

These visual cells stain rather easily, especially in the region of their inner segments. It is easy to establish the fact, well known to histologists, that the lizard retina contains no rods. Furthermore, in good sections it is possible to demonstrate clearly the double cones which have been described in the reptilian retina by M. Schultze, Hoffman, Ranvier, and others.

THE LAYER OF THE VISUAL NUCLEI

If the lizard retina is treated according to the usual techniques (hardening in alcohol or Müller's solution (dichromate), embedding in celloidin, staining with Grenarcher carmine, etc.), three rows of nuclei in the visual cell nuclear layer can be recognized. The outer and the middle rows contain the cone nuclei, while the inner row contains the displaced bipolar cells (Plate III, Fig. 3, *c*).

Nuclei of the Straight Cones

The nuclei of the straight cones are arranged in two rows. The first or outer row is composed of oval nuclei which are situated directly below the outer limiting membrane. The second or inner row contains more elongated elliptical nuclei. A very thin layer of protoplasm, which appears coffee brown or light brown, surrounds the nucleus. A thick trunk arises from the upper pole and is continuous with the inner segment of the cone. A thin fiber arises from the lower pole of the cell and terminates within the outer plexiform layer with a conical swelling. Four or five delicate fibrils emerge from the base of this swelling. After a short, radiating, and horizontal course, these fibrils end freely in a small knob (Plate III, Fig. 2).

Nuclei of the Diagonal Cones

These have an elongated nucleus which lies directly below the outer limiting membrane. Their lower pole sends out a very long, fine fiber which, on changing its direction, forms a bow with a lateral concavity. It then terminates in the inner part of the outer plexiform layer with a conical swelling which is nearly horizontal. Thus, it lies deeper than the feet of the common or straight cones (Plate III, Fig. 1, *c*). In this way the outer plexiform layer is divided into two superimposed strata or plexuses: The first or outer stratum is composed of the fibers which originate from the straight cones and the clusters of certain bipolar cells, whereas the second or inner stratum is composed of the filaments of the diagonal cones and the upper clusters of certain other bipolar cells.

Double Cones

I have succeeded in staining several pairs of these cones (Plate III, Fig. 1, *d*). Each of the two cells has its own nucleus and an independent descending fiber. The terminal swellings of both fibers, however, do not end at the same level. Usually the fiber whose nucleus lies higher sends its end-piece to the outer sublayer of the outer plexiform layer, while the fiber which arises from the other nucleus extends to the inner sublayer of the outer plexiform layer. Thus, it follows that each individual cell of the pair very probably makes contact with a different type of bipolar cell.

Finally, to be complete, I must mention that a few of the cone nuclei exhibit a striation of light and dark bands. Their significance is unclear (Plate III, Fig. 1, *e*).

Displaced Bipolar Cells

These are the outer basal cells of Ranvier[1] which this author studied particularly in the Gecko. (See Plate III, Fig. 7, f, h, g.) Hoffmann[2] described them in the tortoise and first demonstrated their continuity with a Landolt club. In the lizard these cells have the same characteristics as in the frog, except that they are much bigger and are not situated so deep as those of the frog. Their body is fusiform and sometimes also spheroidal (Fig. 7, h). Two processes arise from their two poles: The ascending one is none other than the Landolt club; the descending one terminates in the inner plexiform layer as a free, flattened arborization. At the level of the outer plexiform layer, the descending trunk gives off several short horizontal branches which end freely. Sometimes the ascending branch is absent, or it appears shorter than usual and does not reach the outer limiting membrane (Fig. 7, g). I cannot say whether this is the true state of things, or whether it is because of incomplete staining.

The same observations can be made if the tissue is treated according to the Ehrlich method, although not as distinctly. Methylene blue is especially effective in staining the displaced bipolar cells; on the other hand, it leaves the fibers and the end-feet of the cones unstained.

OUTER PLEXIFORM LAYER

Three types of elements make contact in the outer plexiform layer: the end-feet of both the straight and the diagonal cones, the ascending clusters of both the common and the displaced bipolar cells, and the protoplasmic ramifications of the horizontal cells. As was mentioned above, the outer plexiform layer can be subdivided as: an outer stratum containing the fibers of the straight cones and the upper terminal clusters of certain bipolars, and an inner stratum containing mainly the end-feet of the diagonal cones and another type of bipolar cell which lies deeper.*

---

* The arborization of the horizontal cells, especially those with a brush-shaped upper cluster, appear to contribute to both strata. (1892 edition)

HORIZONTAL CELL LAYER

Horizontal cells of the reptilian retina are rarely stained. Therefore, I have not been able to investigate adequately the extent to which there are homologies between the reptilian horizontal cells and the batrachian and teleost horizontal cells. The most frequent cell types which I encountered in my preparations were the brush-shaped cells ("cellules en brosse") and the stellate cells ("cellules étoilées") (Plate III, Fig. 7, *j, m*).

The Brush-shaped Cells

These are very similar to my inner horizontal cells in the frog and also to the subreticular brush-shaped cells in the bird. (See Fig. 7, *j*.) Their cell body is cuboidal or hemispherical, and it gives off a large number of short, ascending branches from its upper surface. These fibers reach the most superficial part of the outer plexiform layer, where they come into contact with the end-feet of the straight cones. A delicate fiber stems from the lateral portion of the cell body of each brush-shaped cell, and very often, also from a protoplasmic branch. The fiber courses horizontally, and from time to time, gives off short ascending spines which end in a small swelling (Plate III, Fig. 7, *j*). This fiber is probably an axis cylinder whose destination is still unknown to me. Nevertheless, if an analogy may be drawn, I am inclined to think that these nerve processes end at a rather considerable distance in the same plexiform layer with a free terminal ramification. As I will describe later, a very similar axis cylinder in the bird retina follows this type of course. It may be that their end-branches are certain ascending arborizations which are sometimes found in the outer plexiform layer of the lizard retina; such fine horizontal fibers do terminate in the middle of this region (Plate III, Fig. 1, *x*).

Flat Stellate Cells

I have observed these cells with the methylene blue stain. (See Plate III, Fig. 7, *m*.) They have a semilunar shape when viewed from the side. Diverging branches arise from their upper and lateral surfaces, which ascend diagonally to the outer plexiform layer where they appear to terminate after a few divisions. Their axis cylinder has its origin on one side of the cell and courses horizontally between neighboring cells of the same type. I do not yet know where it ends. It seems to me that the protoplasmic branches of these cells do not extend as high in the outer plexiform layer as those of the brush-shaped cells. They might then serve to establish connections among the diagonal cones, whereas the other cells would make connections with the straight cones.*

BIPOLAR CELL LAYER

The bipolar cells of the reptile are almost identical with those found in the frog and bird retina. The results of my research are in complete agreement with those of Dogiel on the bipolar cells of the tortoise. I must, however, add certain minor details.

As I did in the description of the batrachian retina, it is useful at first to distinguish two types of bipolar cells in the reptilian retina: the small or inner bipolar cells, and the large or outer bipolar cells.

A. The Small Bipolar Cells

These are more numerous. They have an oval or fusiform cell body (Plate III, Fig. 1, o) with two processes extending from it, an ascending one and a descending one.

The ascending process is significantly thicker than the descending one. It ascends along a more or less tortuous course to the outer plexiform layer, where it breaks up into a cluster of fine fibers which spread horizontally. Usually, after a short horizontal or diagonal course, one of the branches of the cluster follows a vertical course and forms a Landolt club (Plate III, Fig. 1, s). As we know, this club ends as a small swelling whose tip reaches the outer part of the outer limiting membrane. The other processes of the cluster, which are usually very short and may sometimes number no more than three or four, terminate freely with a knob within the outer plexiform layer. It is not

---

* This hypothesis is a fact demonstrated by my subsequent investigations. (1933 edition)

unusual to see these processes winding their way upward after taking a horizontal course of variable extent, and finally making contact with the basilar swellings of the straight cones.

The descending process generally follows a diagonal course at the level of the so-called inner nuclear layer. As soon as it has arrived at the inner plexiform layer, however, it turns in a vertical direction and ends in one of the sublayers of this zone with a short, varicose, and flat arborization. Just as in the batrachian retina, distinctions can be made on the basis of the number of terminal arborizations. There are (a) bipolars which possess only a single lower arborization (Plate III, Fig. 1, *q*), and (b) bipolars whose descending trunk forms several superimposed arborizations. These spread out at the level of the concentric plexuses formed by the ganglion cells and amacrine cells (Plate III, Fig. 1, *r*). The final arborization, i.e. the branch which lies deepest, very often extends into the lowest part of the fifth sublayer and may come into direct contact with the upper surface of the ganglion cells.

B. The Large Bipolars

These cells correspond exactly to the large bipolar cells of the frog. They have an oval body and lie directly below the outer plexiform layer (Plate III, Fig. 1, *p*). Their nucleus is fairly large, but it is very rare to find them completely stained with chromium-silver because of the rather considerable layer of protoplasm surrounding it. The upper terminal cluster is composed of a few branches which arise directly from the cell body, branch repeatedly, and finally end in a nodule. Most of the terminal fibrils give off ascending spines which terminate with a swelling among the end-feet of the cones. There are no Landolt clubs, or if they are present, I have never been able to stain them. The descending trunk has the same characteristics as that of the common bipolar cells, although it seems to me that the final arborization extends preferentially into the fifth sublayer (Plate III, Fig. 1, *p*).

Regarding the connections between both types of bipolar cells and the cones, it seems probable to me that the large bipolars, i.e. those whose upper terminal cluster reaches the outer part of the outer plexiform layer, have a special connection with the straight cones. On the other hand, the common bipolars, i.e. those whose upper terminal cluster is flattened and extends into a somewhat deeper region of the outer plexiform layer, come into contact with the diagonal cones. However, such relationships are not the only possible ones, since the clusters of the bipolar cells in reptiles are not strictly confined to definite strata, as is the case for the teleost fish and birds. The relationships described above are probably only the predominant ones for each type of bipolar cell.

AMACRINE CELL LAYER

A. Nerve Cells or Dogiel Cells

These cells have a mitral shape and horizontal protoplasmic processes which spread in the first sublayer of the inner plexiform layer. They have an axis cylinder process which, as Dogiel has shown, disappears into the optic nerve fiber layer (Plate III, Fig. 5, *e*).

B. Amacrine Cells

The amacrine cells of the tortoise have been described by Dogiel. His description, however, is so brief that it is difficult to get a precise idea of the quantity and shape of these interesting cells. Dogiel[3] wrote: "The spongioblasts are somewhat larger than the bipolar cells and are located at the outer edge of the neurospongium. Three or four processes originate from the lower surface of the cell. These processes divide several times and anastomose with the neighboring spongioblasts, thus forming a tightly-meshed nerve net in the inner layers of the neurospongium."

After examining Figures 4 and 5 of Plate III, in which I have shown the main forms of amacrine cells, the reader may easily judge the great superiority of the chromium-silver staining method of Golgi, as compared to the Ehrlich method which Dogiel uses exclusively. Similarly, it is easy to become convinced that anastomoses are completely lacking between the branches of the neighboring elements. Furthermore, as I have established in the entire range of vertebrates, each level or sublayer of the inner plexiform layer receives the arborizations of specific spongioblasts.

1. Diffuse Amacrine Cells

These cells are most probably those described by Dogiel as spongioblasts, since they stain especially well with methylene blue (Plate III, Fig. 4, *a, i*; Fig. 5, *a*). Just as I noted in the frog, these cells are small and pyriform. Their descending trunk soon divides into twisted branches which have several short and very varicose collateral extensions. The entire arborization thus formed fills the greater part of the thickness of the inner plexiform layer, although most of the branches tend to be concentrated in the fifth sublayer.

On the basis of the extent of the terminal ramification, two varieties of diffuse amacrine cells can be distinguished: (a) those cells whose main branches take a horizontal course at the level of the first sublayer before descending (Plate III, Fig. 4, *i*) and (b) those cells whose processes arise from a descending trunk and run at an acute angle to their termination which lies below (Plate III, Fig. 4, *a* and Fig. 5, *a*).*

B. Stratified Amacrine Cells

1. Stratified Amacrine Cells of the First Sublayer

Up to now I have succeeded in finding only one type of cell in this layer. They are semilunar in shape and have very long, radiating processes which arise from their lower surface and extend horizontally (Plate III, Fig. 4, *f*).

2. Amacrine Cells of the Second Sublayer

Here it is relatively easy to distinguish three varieties of cell: the giant amacrine cells with stout branches, the amacrine cells with fine, radiating arborizations, and the amacrine cells with dense and compact clusters.

(a) *The giant amacrine cells.* These cells are quite remark-

---

* The primary and secondary extensions of these cells are often covered with small spines or collateral branches which end in a varicosity. (1892 edition)

able. Their cell body is pyriform and more or less irregularly shaped (Plate III, Fig. 4, *e*). Their descending trunk forms a magnificent star of thick, horizontal branches upon their arrival at the level of the second sublayer. The diverging branches retain their original thickness over a considerable distance, but they suddenly become fine and flat. From that point on, they look very much like an axis cylinder (Plate III, Fig. 4, *m* and Plate IV, Fig. 2, *b*). The processes then run for an enormous distance (more than 0.7 mm) without branching. It should also be noted that they increase slightly in thickness before they terminate with a small swelling. These extraordinary cells are represented as viewed from above in Plate IV, Figure 2 and in profile in Plate II, Figure 4, *e*.

(b) *Amacrine cells with fine stellate clusters* ("panache fin et étoilé"). In the future I will refer to these cells as amacrine cells with radial clusters ("à panache rayonnant"). They have the characteristics of analogous cells which I described in the teleost fish and the frog, so that I do not need to repeat their description here. I would like to add, however, that the radiating fibers are extraordinarily fine and that they terminate with a varicose terminal knob at the level of the second sublayer (Plate III, Fig. 5, *h*). It can be seen that these fibers increase measurably in thickness again, at a certain distance before they terminate, and that their varicosities become larger. This is especially true for the longer fibers. (Some can be followed for more than 1 mm.)

(c) *Amacrine cells with short, compact clusters* (Plate III, Fig. 5, *b*, *c*). These are pyriform and have a foot-piece that turns down and may form either a single slender trunk or several divisions; sometimes an abrupt division of the single trunk may also occur. The terminal arborization lies in the second sublayer and is composed of winding, varicose branches so close to one another that it is often difficult to follow the course of each individual branch. Based on their size, these elements can be classified as small (Plate III, Fig. 5, *c*) or middle-sized (Plate III, Fig. 5, *b*) cells.

In order to be complete, I must mention yet another type of giant cell, having a mitral or semilunar shape, which I have encountered exclusively in preparations treated by Dogiel's method (Plate III, Fig. 7, n). Two single, thick processes extend from the opposite sides of the cell body and then descend diagonally to ramify in the second sublayer.

3. Amacrine Cells of the Third Sublayer

Three varieties of such cells can be seen: cells with fibrillar, radiating arborizations; cells with short, winding arborizations; and giant cells.

(a) *Cells with radiating ramifications.* These are larger than the corresponding cells of the second sublayer. They have an arborization whose terminal fibrils are straight and which are of considerable length (Plate III, Fig. 4, b, g).

(b) *Cells with short arborizations.* These cells are pyriform and rather large. They send out short, horizontal, varicose, and moderately-branched ramifications at the level of the third sublayer (Plate III, Fig. 4, h).

(c) *Giant cells.* These cells may just be the same cells described immediately above, although they can be distinguished by their exaggerated dimensions (Plate III, Fig. 5, f). In any case, these cells are consistently observed in all vertebrates, although their dimensions are greatest in reptiles. The cells drawn in Plate III, Fig. 5 (from an adult lizard) are representative of this cell type. They are pyriform and have a cell body so large that its upper part extends almost as far as the outer plexiform layer. The very thick trunk of this cell breaks up into a flat, irregular stellate arborization with thick varicose branches.

In a very young *Lacerta agilis* I have found a few cells of this type with an arborization which was amazingly regular and very extensive. In addition, in an especially well stained horizontal section, it can be seen that all of the terminal ramifications go only to one level, where they come into contact with one another and are tightly interlaced.

4. Amacrine Cells of the Fourth Sublayer

Apart from the absence of the giant type of cell, the cells of this sublayer are entirely similar to those of the preceding layer. A small type of cell whose descending trunk forms an arborization of very fine radiating filaments can also be seen (Plate III, Fig. 4, d) here. Rather large cell bodies can also be found; their descending trunk breaks up into a cluster of thick varicose fibers which ramify repeatedly and are very dense.

5. Amacrine Cells of the Fifth Sublayer

I have found arborizations in this sublayer which are related to two cell types commonly encountered: (a) cells with a gnarled, loose, and relatively short tuft (Plate III, Fig. 4, c), (b) cells with a filamentous, radiating terminal cluster whose fibrils spread enormously in the deepest region of the fifth sublayer without ever dividing (Plate III, Fig. 5, d).

Bistratified amacrine cells. In this category I place those multipolar cells which are hemispherical and lie directly above the inner plexiform layer (Plate III, Fig. 5, g). A few horizontal branches arise from the contours of their cell body. A short distance from the cell body they suddenly take a vertical course and then form a plexus of very long, slender fibers in the fifth sublayer. Also, several branches of these cells ramify in the first two sublayers; these branches arise either from the main processes or from the cell body itself. Such cells can also be found in mammals (Plate V, Fig. 7, C) and frogs (Plate II, Fig. 3, G), but with some modifications.

THE GANGLION CELL LAYER

The retina of the reptile is very rich in varieties of ganglion cells. Among these are found some whose protoplasmic processes are so fine that the strongest objective must be used for distinguishing and resolving them. Others show multilayered arborizations of admirable form and elegance. In general the reptile can be considered to be the vertebrate in which the amacrine cells and ganglion cells have reached their highest degree of evolution and perfection.

A. Single-layered Cells

I have found single-layered cells in only a few sublayers, but perhaps I have not been successful in staining them wherever they occur. The cells which I did encounter most frequently are the following:

1. Small Cells Which Ramify in the Fourth Sublayer

These cells (Plate III, Fig. 5, C and Fig. 6, D, F) are evidently the most abundant of their kind; they correspond exactly to the small cells of the fourth sublayer described for the teleost fish and the frog. They have a pyriform cell body with an ascending process that divides initially into three or four branches and then breaks up into a flat terminal arborization which lies entirely within the fourth sublayer. This arborization consists of an extraordinarily large number of entangled, varicose branches which are very close to one another. When viewed in profile, these arborizations look like a coffee-brown granular mass. The group of all these arborizations forms an almost continuous granular line parallel with the surface of the retina in the fourth sublayer. I believe that these cells have an axis cylinder, but as yet I have not been able to stain them.*

2. Ganglion Cells of the Second Sublayer

These cells (Plate III, Fig. 6, I) are giant pyriform cells which have a very robust ascending process. After this process has reached the second sublayer, it breaks up into a very flat ramification with extraordinarily thick and entangled branches.

3. Ganglion Cells of the First Sublayer

To this group belong certain middle-sized multipolar cells whose numerous delicate processes initially follow a horizontal course within the web of the fourth sublayer. (See Plate III, Fig. 5, D.) Then they ascend, travelling through the entire inner plexiform layer. Ultimately they form a tightly-packed plexus of fine, varicose branches in the upper portion of this layer. Besides these direct branches, there are several fine, ascending collateral branches which originate from the horizontal portion of these trunks, and which also contribute to the formation of this plexus.

---

*These are displaced amacrine cells which have no axis cylinder. (1933 edition)

B. Multilayered Cells

1. Cells of the Second, Third, and Fourth Sublayers

Of all the multilayered cells, these are the most abundant. In the reptile they are truly remarkable in their regular and elegant shape. Two varieties can be distinguished: One is thin, and the other is stout. Aside from this difference, the two types of cells are very similar (Plate III, Fig. 6, *H, C*).

When these cells are multipolar, the cell body is semilunar, and when they have only one ascending process, the cell body is pyriform or pyramidal. The single trunk, or the various ascending trunks, bifurcate once or twice during the first part of their course. When they have reached the fourth sublayer, almost all of them course horizontally and form their first plexus of tightly twisted branches.* A large number of fine and virtually straight branches ascend at a right angle from this plexus to the second sublayer. There they branch again and form a second plexus of short, twisted, and extremely varicose filaments. On their passage through the third sublayer a few of these ascending fibers send out small, twisted, varicose collateral branches, whose intertwining forms a loose intermediate plexus.

2. Cells of the First and Fifth Sublayers

In this category I have included certain multipolar and fusiform cells, most of whose protoplasmic branches are arranged in a very loose plexus in the region of the ganglion cell layer, i.e. in the fifth sublayer. A few of their branches divide, however, and participate in the formation of a plexus in the first sublayer (Plate III, Fig. 6, *G*).

3. Multilayered Ganglion Cells with Fine Granular Arborizations

These are small multilayered cells which are very remarkable in that their protoplasmic branches are extremely fine (the most delicate fibers I know of). They form very dense granular plex-

---

* The branches are angular at the point of origin of the secondary branches. (1892 edition)

uses which are much thicker than those ordinarily encountered in the sublayers of the inner plexiform layer (Plate III, Fig. 5, A, B and Fig. 6, E).

I have classified these cells into two different types, based on the location and extent of their terminal arborizations: cells whose diffuse terminal plexus spreads in the third and fourth sublayers (Plate III, Fig. 5, A), and cells whose terminal plexus is concentrated mainly at the levels of the third, fourth, and the upper half of the fifth sublayers (Plate III, Fig. 5, B and Fig. 6, E). In all of these cells the plexus is composed of progressively finer granules, the more peripherally it is located.

C. Diffuse Ganglion Cells

I have found only one diffuse ganglion cell (Plate III, Fig. 6, A) which is large, semilunar, and multipolar. It has ascending protoplasmic branches which ramify throughout the entire thickness of the inner plexiform layer without exhibiting any tendency to form a horizontal plexus.

In Plate III, Figure 6, B, I have shown another cell which might be included in this category. I noted, however, that most of its protoplasmic branches ramify in the fifth sublayer, and only a few seem to end in the first sublayer. In their fusiform shape, these cells resemble those which I saw in the fifth sublayer of the inner plexiform layer of the teleost fish and mammals.

Autochthonous Ganglion Cells of the Inner Plexiform Layer

I have succeeded in staining a few oval or mitral-shaped cells whose ascending processes arborize in the first sublayer (Plate III, Fig. 4, *j*). A nerve process arises from the lower pole of their cell body and extends to the optic nerve fiber layer. It is clear that we are not dealing here with an amacrine cell of the inner plexiform layer, as is the case in the mammalian retina. Rather, we have a displaced ganglion cell, which belongs to that class of ganglion cells whose protoplasmic branches form a single horizontal plexus.

In the description of the amacrine cells and ganglion cells I have assumed that there are five sublayers or levels of arborization in the inner plexiform layer. This division into five plexuses is not absolute: In the space between the fourth and fifth sublayers (which is very large in the reptile) and likewise between the second and third sublayers, protoplasmic ramifications of the amacrine and ganglion cells can be found. These appear to form two other plexuses which are more or less well defined. The five plexuses which I have described are those plexuses whose staining and study is relatively easy, probably because of their considerable development and the large number of arborizations which they contain. In addition it appears that the five plexuses extend throughout the retina, whereas intercalated plexuses are found only in the regions of maximal thickness of the retina.

OPTIC NERVE FIBER LAYER

By staining the retina with methylene blue it can be determined that the fibers of this layer are arranged in bundles which diverge from the optic disk. These bundles are separated by the descending processes of the Müller or epithelial cells. Every bundle contains two or three thick fibers and a considerable number of smaller fine fibers.

In young lizards I occasionally observed fine collateral ascending fibrils which, upon reaching the lower portion of the inner plexiform layer, ramified and terminated freely (Plate III, Fig. 7, *t*). I cannot determine, however, the type of fiber which this collateral branch is nor the significance of the fact that I never found them in adult animals or in higher vertebrates.

EPITHELIAL CELLS

Except for several minor details, these cells are entirely similar to those found in the bird retina (Plate VI, Fig. 3). They are distinguished only by the fact that their descending cluster has far fewer fibrils in the region between the nucleus of the Müller cell and the level of the amacrine cells. In the bird there are twenty to thirty descending fibrils in a cluster, whereas there are only four to eight such fibrils in the reptile. In their passage through the inner plexiform layer, these fibrils send out short varicose collateral branches which look like curly down-feathers.

These downy processes disappear again at the level of the main plexuses, or at least they decrease significantly in number. On the other hand, they appear more numerous in the region surrounding these plexuses.

The divisions of the lower part of the Müller fibers in reptiles and birds has been mentioned by a few histologists, notably Schiefferdecker.[4] But all the details of the epithelial cell become evident only by staining with chromium-silver.

If the optic nerve is treated with chromium-silver, a large number of stellate neuroglial cells similar to those seen in the frog can be observed among the individual bundles of the nerve. In contrast, I have never seen these cells in the optic nerve fiber layer of the retina.

REFERENCES

1. Ranvier, L.: *Traité technique d'histologie.* Paris, 1872-1875, p. 961.
2. Hoffmann, C.: Zur Anatomie der Retina. I. Über den Bau der Retina bei Amphibien und Reptilien. *Niederl. Arch. f. Zool.*, 1876 (3), 12.
3. Dogiel, A.: Über das Verhalten der nervösen Element in der Retina der Ganoiden, Reptilien, Vögel, and Säugetiere. *Anat. Anz.*, 1888 (3), 138.
4. Schiefferdecker, P.: Studien zur vergleichenden Histologie der Retina. *Arch. f. mikrosk. Anat.*, 1886 (28), 305-396.

Chapter VI

THE RETINA OF BIRDS

SEVERAL years ago I published a communication on the avian retina which contained the findings I had obtained using the rapid Golgi method on various species of birds.[1] Therefore, in the present report I will be very brief on this subject, limiting myself to calling attention to a few new facts. The results previously communicated will be mentioned only as they may correct or complete the story for the bird retina. My earlier efforts were concentrated on many diverse species, but recently I have been concerned mainly with the retina of gallinaceous birds.

THE VISUAL CELL LAYER

Just as in the other vertebrates, I have observed that in birds the inner segments of the rods and cones are stained more easily with chromium-silver than is the outer segment. From time to time, though, visual cells can be found which are completely stained.

In successful preparations it is easy to recognize that there are two types of cones in the bird retina, just as Hoffmann described At the level of the inner segment one type is much enlarged, whereas the other is very slender and delicate and can hardly be distinguished from the rods.

From the interesting observations of M. Schultze, we know that diurnal birds have a very small number of rods, whereas nocturnal birds have a great number of them. Cones, however, are not absent in the nocturnal birds, but are found only in small numbers.

The colored oil droplets of the cones, which have been described by Schultze,[2] Schwalbe,[3] Krause,[4] Dobrowsky,[5] Hoffmann,[6] Beauregard,[7] et al. are not revealed with the chromium-silver method, which stains them black along with the remaining protoplasm of the visual cell. In cones which are not stained the osmic acid contained in the osmium-dichromate mixture colors the oil droplets dark-grey, so that no colors can be discerned.

THE LAYER OF THE VISUAL CELL NUCLEI

This layer contains four types of granules or visual cell bodies: the cell bodies of the rods, the cell bodies of the straight cones, the cell bodies of the diagonal cones, and the cell bodies of the double-cones.

A. The Nuclei of the Rods

In general these nuclei lie in the lower half of the outer nuclear layer. An ascending and a descending process arises from each of the poles of the cell, both of which are remarkably thick. The descending process is very short, enlarges gradually, and finally terminates in a flat surface. Fine lateral filaments arise from the contours of this surface, and they extend into the outermost stratum of the outer plexiform zone (Plate IV, Fig. 6, c).

In the passerine birds (sparrow, green finch, chaffinch), after taking a short and nearly horizontal course at the level of the upper stratum of this zone, these basilar filaments descend obliquely to ramify in the region of the horizontal cell layer. The terminal branches extend over a rather wide region in the outer plexiform zone, but those that arise from the cones are very short and branch only slightly (Plate IV, Fig. 9, a).

B. The Nuclei of the Straight Cones

In gallinaceous birds these cells lie directly below the outer limiting membrane. They are oval and have a delicate descending fiber which terminates with a conical swelling in the middle stratum of the outer plexiform layer. Radiating filaments course horizontally from the lower surface of this swelling (Plate IV, Fig. 6, b). Occasionally a few terminal swellings of the cones may be found lying at the upper boundary of the outer plexiform layer. The fibrils which arise from these cone swellings, however, descend and distribute within the middle stratum of the outer plexiform layer, in much the same way as those from the other straight cones (Plate IV, Fig. 8, h).

C. The Nuclei of the Diagonal Cones

These are distinguished from the nuclei of the straight cones by the orientation of their descending fibers and the manner in which they terminate. They have a very long fiber which bends more and more to the side during its course. When this fiber finally reaches the outer plexiform layer, it is lying almost completely horizontally. Hence, the terminal swelling is diagonally or even horizontally oriented and extends into the deepest stratum (the inner stratum) of the outer plexiform layer. At this point it gives rise to numerous fine branches which interweave with those arising from neighboring swellings. Sometimes separate collateral branches arise from the convex side of the descending fiber in its course. Such collateral branches end in the same manner (Plate IV, Fig. 8, c and Fig. 6, e).

I have found the longest obliquely-descending fiber in the retina of the turkey (Plate IV, Fig. 6, e). Here there are fibers which course obliquely through the outer plexiform layer for more than 0.08 mm. Along its horizontal course four to six collateral branches are given off and ramify in the region of the inner stratum of the outer plexiform layer.

Lastly, there are diagonal cones whose terminal swellings lie on the other side of the outer plexiform layer, i.e. within the horizontal cell layer. There they form a roundish or cuboidal swelling (Plate IV, Fig. 8, d). It is very interesting that the basilar filaments of these cones ascend from this swelling and are distributed within the same level as the basilar filaments which arise from the other diagonal cones, namely in the inner stratum of the outer plexiform layer.

D. The Double Cones

These cones often stain very beautifully, thereby making it possible to see that both cones are in intimate contact with one another yet also independent of one another, as many histologists have already described. Each member of the pair has a different-sized nucleus, the larger of the two having a lateral indentation in which the smaller one is partially embedded. The two descending fibers are of unequal lengths, a characteristic I described previously in the reptiles. The fiber which usually arises from the larger nucleus descends into the deepest stratum of the outer plexiform layer and forms a very voluminous swelling there. The other fiber extends to the middle or even the most external stratum of the outer plexiform zone. Delicate filaments proceed from the terminal swelling of both cone fibers, and they arrange themselves within the corresponding plexus of the outer plexiform layer (Plate IV, Fig. 6, d and Fig. 8, f).

As noted earlier, the diagonal cones are a consistent finding in the retina of frogs, reptiles, and birds. This is also true for the double cones.

Do the diagonal cones represent visual cells which are physiologically different from the straight cones, or are we dealing here with only a topographic difference, the purpose of which is to increase the contact surface with the bipolar cells without losing the individuality of the impulses which they conduct?

At present it is impossible to answer these questions; we can only conjecture. There is one fact, though, which supports the idea that the diagonal cones have a particular function. We know that in the frog retina almost all the oblique nuclei are connected with certain specialized rods. These are the green rods (the club-shaped rods of Schwalbe), which are completely distinguishable from the common, or red, rods. If we suppose that the oblique nuclei of reptiles and birds have a similar functional specificity, we might think that in these animals the diagonal nuclei are continuous with receptors having an oil droplet of a particular color, or some other morphological characteristic which is yet unknown to us.

Similarly the equally fascinating problem of the physiological significance of the double cones remains obscure. We can assert only that each member of the cone pair has its own individual function. This assertion is supported by the following facts: Each of the two descending fibers extends its basilar fibers into a different plexus of the plexiform layer and probably makes contact with different bipolar cells. It is even possible that there is a slightly different luminous sensitivity for each of the two cones, as was suggested by M. Schultze,[8] and by Hoffmann.[9] Some time ago these investigators demonstrated that there is an oil droplet in the smaller of the two cones which is of a slightly different color from that of the principal cone.

I have never found displaced bipolar cells (Ranvier's "cellules basales externes," Krause's compensatory cells) in the bird. I believe that they are totally absent here, because I could not find them in retinal sections stained with carmine or aniline dyes. Schiefferdecker is of the same opinion.

Finally at this time I would like to mention a fact which I described in an earlier report but which has been substantiated by more recent work. I have found that the rods of nocturnal birds (screech owl, *Bubo bubo*) have almost the same shape and position as mammalian rods. They also terminate as a nodule with no basilar filament in the outermost part of the outer plexiform layer.[1] The terminal spherule is surrounded by the ascending clusters of certain bipolar cells. The cones, whose pedicles have the same general appearance, descend more deeply than the rods and make contact with other bipolar cells which have flat clusters and also lie deeper.

THE OUTER PLEXIFORM LAYER

As stated previously, the outer plexiform layer is composed of three concentric layers or plexuses in gallinaceous birds:* (a) The outer stratum is formed by the basilar fibrils of the rods and the upper terminal clusters of certain bipolar cells. (b) The middle or intermediate stratum is composed of terminal fibers of the straight cones and the ascending clusters of a different type of bipolar cell. (c) The inner stratum consists of fibrils which arise from the diagonal cones and the upper terminal clusters of certain other bipolars. We should mention also the protoplasmic branches of the horizontal cells, which appear to be spread into all three of these strata and also the terminal branches of the axis cylinders of these cells. It is possible from the above to get an idea of the extreme complexity of the outer plexiform layer of the bird retina. Moreover, I believe that the

---

* One could also say here that just as in the inner plexiform layer the outer plexiform layer can be divided into so many "sublayers." However, this would easily lead to confusion, since the bipolar cells project into both the inner and the outer plexiform layers. Therefore, the word "sublayer" shall be used always to denote one of the concentric plexuses in the *inner* plexiform layer. In the outer plexiform layer, where the end-feet of the visual cells meet with the upper clusters of the bipolar cells, the individual layers of ramification will be translated as "concentric layers" or "strata." (Greeff's note)

construction of this layer may be somewhat modified in different species of birds, especially in small birds.

HORIZONTAL CELL LAYER

Brush-shaped Cells ("Cellules en Brosse")

I have described the existence of this type of cell (Plate IV, Fig. 6, h) in an earlier work on the bird retina. The brush-shaped cells have numerous short protoplasmic processes. As they ascend through the outer plexiform layer, they resemble the bristles of a thick brush whose fibers extend to the most external margin of the outer plexiform layer. Very often the filaments of these cells can be seen to be arranged in separate clusters. Two or three large gaps are left between these clusters, into which the pedicles of the straight cones are inserted (Plate IV, Fig. 6, h and Fig. 8, i).

The axis cylinder of these cells extends horizontally beneath the outer plexiform layer and can usually be traced for a distance of 0.30 to 0.40 mm. It terminates with a dense flat ramification whose branches have the appearance of diverging spines and whose sides are elongated in the form of slightly ascending spines. Although I am not entirely certain, I believe that these arborizing plaques spread directly beneath the feet of the straight cones.*

Stellate Horizontal Cells

In addition to the horizontal cells described above, another type of cell can be found in this layer. These are flat stellate cells with extensions which are longer but not as dense. (See

---

* Previously I noticed these peculiar terminal swellings beneath the cone feet only in gallinaceous birds. Recently, however, in the sparrow and green finch, I have also seen flat terminal ramifications at this particular location. I am not yet sure, though, that they are identical to that which I described in the gallinaceous birds or whether they represent a special type of arborization, e.g. the terminal swelling of the axis cylinder of the stellate horizontal cells. These are rather thick horizontal fibers which are displaced some distance from the outer plexiform layer and can be traced over a large area. Before forming their terminal arborization they ascend in a bow, decrease in diameter, and finally dissolve into a short, flat, diffuse arborization whose numerous end-branches appear to ascend between the end-feet of the visual cells and terminate in a knob. These terminal arborizations are more extensive and fully developed than those seen in the gallinaceous birds. (1894 edition)

Plate IV, Fig. 8, *j* and Fig. 6, *f*.) They end freely in the uppermost portion of the outer plexiform layer. At first their large axis cylinder descends, but it then takes a horizontal course and becomes progressively thinner as it runs for a considerable distance beneath the outer plexiform zone. I cannot be sure of the mode of termination, however, since my observations are as yet incomplete. In Figure 7, *a*, Plate IV, I have drawn two stellate cells in a surface view, as I saw them in a horizontal section through the chicken retina. It should be noted that the axis cylinder does not give rise to any fine collateral branches throughout its entire length.

THE BIPOLAR CELL LAYER

I have a few more things to add to my description of these cells which appeared in the 1889 *Anatomische Anzeiger*, and likewise to Dogiel's (1888) description.

The bipolar cells can be classified into two groups: (a) the outer bipolar cells, which lie below the outer plexiform layer, and (b) the inner or small bipolar cells, which occupy the remainder of the bipolar cell layer.

The ascending cluster of the outer bipolar cells (Plate IV, Fig. 8, *n*) is quite fully developed, very extensive, and apparently has no Landolt club. The corresponding cluster of the thin or inner bipolar cells does not take its origin from the cell body, as is the case for the outer bipolar cells. Instead, it arises from the end of an ascending trunk (Plate IV, Fig. 8, *o*, *p*) and is composed of a small number of horizontally-oriented fibrils which lie in one of the three concentric strata of the outer plexiform layer. One of these fibers elongates into a Landolt club (Plate IV, Fig. 8, *l*).

The lower process of the small bipolars often sends out collateral branches at the various sublayers of the inner plexiform layer.* The descending process ends with a varicose ramification, or sometimes it breaks up into two neighboring arborizations (Plate IV, Fig. 8, *s*, *t*). Most of the descending processes extend

---

* The existence of such collateral branches has recently been confirmed by an investigation of Dogiel,[10] but Dogiel has the habit of not citing me. (Cajal's note in the 1894 edition.)

The Retina of Birds

their terminal arborization into the area lying between the fourth and fifth sublayers.

The terminal arborization of the descending processes of the large or outer bipolar cells (Plate IV, Fig. 8, n) appears to occur preferentially in the fifth sublayer; however, I have been successful in staining this terminal ramification only a very few times. Thus, I would not like to say anything definite concerning the location.

AMACRINE CELL LAYER

The cells of this region are almost identical to those seen in the reptilian retina. At the outset, one can distinguish (a) the mitral-shaped nerve cells that were very well described by Dogiel, and (b) the genuine amacrine cells. I should like to add a few details about this second type of cell.

In the bird the amacrine cells form five principal plexuses which are stacked atop one another in the inner plexiform layer. In many areas of the retina, however, more sublayers are found—six or seven. Hence, it is possible to classify the amacrine cells by the numerical order of the inner plexiform sublayer in which they arborize. An exception to this is the nonstratified or diffuse amacrine cells, which comprise a special group.

A. Diffuse Amacrine Cells

These are small, pyriform elements which lie in the upper region of the amacrine cell layer. (See Plate IV, Fig. 8, G, L.) Their descending trunk breaks up as soon as it reaches the inner plexiform layer to form a cluster of delicate, varicose, descending branches with small, rounded ends. Often, in the course of their descent, the branches of this cell ramify and give rise to short, very tortuous varicose branches at the level of one of the sublayers of the inner plexiform zone. This peculiarity gives some cells of this type a multilayered appearance (Plate IV, Fig. 8, L).

When I looked at these cells for the first time, my attention was directed to the delicacy and great number of the descending filaments. These filaments are completely comparable to the extensions of the so-called spider cells ("cellules en araignée," "Spinnenzellen"). For this reason, I called them "neuroglia-shaped spongioblasts" in my first publication, on the supposition that they did in fact represent a variety of neuroglia cell. Since then, however, I have observed these cells in all classes of vertebrates and have examined them minutely. Now I do not hesitate to consider them to be a variety of amacrine cell, which differs from the others by the total absence or incomplete stratification of their descending branches.

B. The Stratified Amacrine Cells

1. Amacrine Cells of the First Sublayer

I have found two types of these cells: (a) small semilunar cells with delicate straight horizontal processes of enormous length, arising from their contours (Plate IV, Fig. 8, A, B); (b) larger cells, which are also semilunar but whose diverging branches are much thicker than those of the first type of cell (Plate IV, Fig. 8, C). The branches of both these cell types spread radially at the outer boundary of the inner plexiform layer and form an extraordinarily rich plexus. Some of the fibers which make up this complicated plexus can be followed over a distance of more than one millimeter. They seem to maintain their individuality and a virtually constant diameter throughout their long course; they are totally independent of other cell processes.

2. Amacrine Cells of the Second Sublayer

I have found the same two cell types here which I have already described in reptiles: (a) small cells with a thin descending trunk which gives off a very dense ramification of short, varicose, fibers in the second sublayer (Plate IV, Fig. 8, D), and (b) larger, pyriform cells with a descending trunk which extends into the second sublayer and breaks up into a magnificent flat stellate ramification. The fine filaments of this ramification are straight and quite long (Plate IV, Fig. 8, E).

3. Amacrine Cells of the Third Sublayer

These are also very similar to those cells seen in the reptilian retina. Two types are found: (a) giant pyriform cells whose very stout lower trunk forms a flat arborization containing only a few, thick, coarse branches (Plate IV, Fig. 8, *M*) and (b) middle-sized multipolar or monopolar cells whose terminal ramifications have very twisted and varicose branches of limited length (Plate IV, Fig. 8, *K*).

Probably there are also amacrine cells in the third sublayer with filamentous radiating branches, since such elements are found in reptiles, frogs, and mammals.

4. Amacrine Cells of the Fourth Sublayer

Here both types of frequently encountered cells are found: (a) the pyriform cells with loose, twisted arborizations which are rather limited in extent (Plate IV, Fig. 8, *J*) and (b) cells with a very straight and delicate trunk which terminates in a magnificent star, whose linear branches are very long and fine (Plate IV, Fig. 8, *N*).

5. Amacrine Cells of the Fifth Sublayer

The same two types of cell occur here as in the fourth sublayer: the type with short, twisted arborizations and the type with long, stellate arborizations (Plate IV, Fig. 8, *I*).*†

---

* This addition was made in order to complete the description of the amacrine cells published in my earlier work. These are elements which are quite striking and very numerous in birds. (See Fig. 4, b). Their pyriform cell body sends out a descending process which terminates in a bouquet of short, thick dendrites. The axis cylinder is large and horizontal, and it arises from the lowest part of the descending process. It proceeds within either the first sublayer of the inner plexiform layer, or to the upper boundary of this zone. After a very long course, it terminates in an extremely varicose and tangled arborization, articulating with a considerable number of descending trunks from ordinary amacrine cells. Ehrlich's method demonstrates that the cell bodies and dendrites of the association amacrine cells are surrounded by the terminal arborizations of exogenous centrifugal fibers. Figures 4 and 5 of the text show the form and connections of these unique cells, and Figure 6 presents the probable course of centrifugal fibers. (1933 edition)

† Sometimes in sparrows amacrine cells can be found having a descending process which forms a horizontal plexus at the level of the second sublayer. Two or more descending branches arise from this plexus and extend to the level of the fourth sublayer, where they ramify anew and form a second plexus. Thus, these cells form two terminal ramifications which are separated from another yet superimposed. (1894 edition)

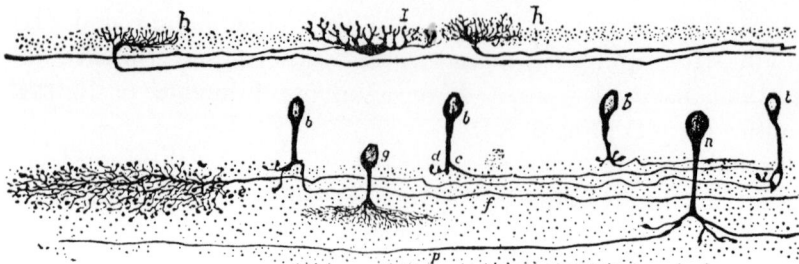

Figure 4. Retina of a passerine bird (green finch). *b* association amacrine cell; *d* rudimentary dendrites of such a cell; *c, f* horizontal axis cylinder; *e* terminal arborization of this fiber; *l* flat horizontal cell; *h, i* horizontal arborization of the axis cylinder of such a cell; *g, n* ordinary amacrine cells.

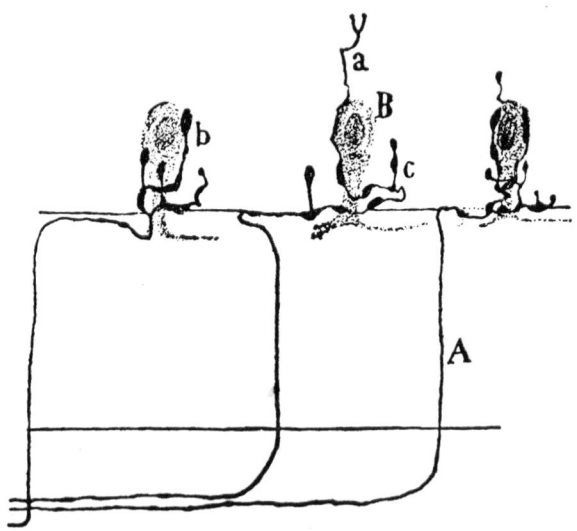

Figure 5. Centrifugal fibers in the retina of the pigeon. Ehrlich-Bethe method. *A* nerve fiber proceeding from the higher nervous center; *B* association amacrine cell enveloped by the ramification of the centrifugal fiber; *a, b, c* varicose terminal arborizations.

The Retina of Birds

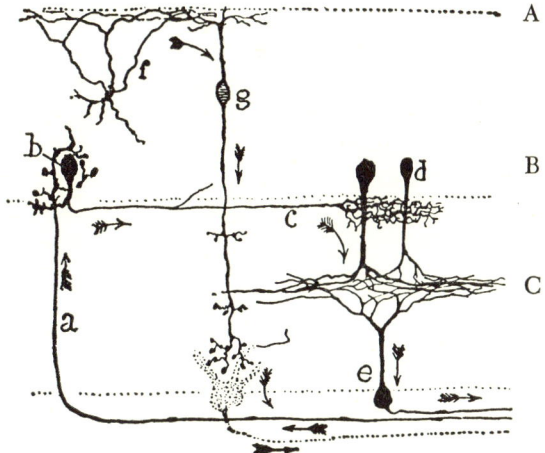

Figure 6. Schema depicting the path of nervous conduction within the system comprised of centrifugal fibers and amacrine cells of association. *A* outer plexiform layer; *B* inner nuclear layer; *C* inner plexiform layer; *a* centrifugal fiber; *b* association amacrine cell; *d* ordinary amacrine cell which makes contact with the arborization *c* of the axon of the association amacrine cell at its trunk; *e* ganglion cell body; *g* bipolar cell. (Retina of a passerine bird)

GANGLION CELL LAYER

A. Single-layered Cells

I have found the following types of cells most frequently in the retina of gallinaceous birds:

1. Giant pyriform cells which form a very gnarled, flat arborization at the level of the first sublayer (Plate V, Fig. 1, *A*).
2. Middle-sized pyriform cells which form a varicose terminal arborization in the second sublayer (Plate V, Fig. 1, *B*).
3. Middle-sized multipolar cells which form a fine arborization in the second sublayer (Plate V, Fig. 1, *D*).
4. Small pyriform cells whose granular and extremely dense arborization lies within the fourth sublayer (Plate V, Fig. 1, *C*). These cells, which are the smallest of the ganglion

cells, correspond to the single-layered cells of the fourth sublayer in fish, reptiles, batrachians, and mammals.*

B. Multilayered Cells

The cells which I found most frequently are the following: (a) multipolar cells which furnish horizontal plexuses to three sublayers, namely to the second, third, and fourth sublayers (Plate V, Fig. 1, G). I will not give a detailed description of these cells since they are entirely similar to those cells which occur in the same sublayers of reptiles. The reader should compare Plate V, Fig. 1, G with Plate III, Fig. 6, C and H. (b) Somewhat smaller multipolar cells with two horizontal plexuses: One plexus has thick branches and lies in the outer part of the fifth sublayer, whereas the other plexus has fine branches and lies in the third sublayer (Plate V, Fig. 1, E). In the reptile there are cells which are very similar to the ones just described, except they have finer branches (Plate III, Fig. 6, E). (c) Small multipolar cells which form three plexuses: one in the fifth sublayer, another in the fourth, and finally, one in the second (Plate V, Fig. 1, F).†

---

* Recently I have succeeded in finding the same type of very small ganglion cells in the sparrow, which despite their delicate, compact terminal arborizations, develop in the third sublayer. Probably such fine arborizations occur in each of the five sublayers and originate from a single-layered ganglion cell. Likewise there are probably such ramifications in each of the sublayers which arise from multilayered ganglion cells. It appears from the above description that it is precisely the avian retina which is the most complicated, with respect to the structure of the inner plexiform layer and the morphology of the spongioblasts and ganglion cells. (1894 edition)

† Besides the ganglion cells mentioned above, it is likely that there are others which will be revealed by further staining attempts. (1892 edition)

These small ganglion cells, whose arborizations are composed of very fine fibrils, occur quite frequently in the retina of sparrows, in fact more frequently than I had initially believed. Recently in the chaffinch and in the green finch, I have found several odd types of multilayered cells with fine terminal branches:

1. Cells whose ascending and usually singular process forms three very delicate plexuses which lie in the fourth, second, and somewhat below the third sublayer.

2. Cells whose ascending trunk divides gradually, thus forming two fine plexuses, the first extending into the fourth sublayer and the second into the second sublayer.

(Continued on next page)

THE OPTIC FIBER LAYER

Here I have been able to confirm certain of my earlier observations. Occasionally it is possible to find certain thick fibers which arise from the optic nerve and penetrate the inner plexiform layer; they then ascend to the level of the amacrine cells. Here they terminate with thick, varicose, and completely freely-ending branches (Plate V, Fig. 1, *a, b, d*). Since the terminal extremities of this branch hardly extend beyond the boundary of the amacrine cell layer (the spongioblasts), it seems quite likely that these centrifugal fibers serve to transmit impulses from the visual centers of the brain to the amacrine cells. The existence of centrifugal fibers was suggested by Monakow[11] on the basis of pathological-anatomical studies.*

(Continued from preceding page)

3. Cells with three plexuses, which probably lie (a) somewhat below the fourth, (b) in the third, and (c) in the first sublayers.

Other cell types were also found. (1894 edition)

Among the passerine birds (sparrow, green finch, chaffinch, linnet, etc.), in addition to the five principal plexuses of the inner plexiform zone, two supernumerary plexuses are found. One is located beneath the fourth sublayer, and the other between the third and second sublayers. Among the gallinaceous birds I have not succeeded in staining these accessory plexuses. (1892 edition)

It would be better to distinguish seven rather than five sublayers in the inner plexiform layer of the bird, for in the thickest parts of the retina a supplementary sublayer can always be found somewhat above the middle portion of the fifth sublayer. A second such layer occurs in the third sublayer a bit above its central portion.

All of these arborizations are exceptionally fine; a dense plexus arises from the numerous fine varicose branches, which can be resolved only with a strong objective. (1894 edition)

* Recently Dogiel[12] has also reported centrifugal fibers in the bird retina, which I myself had described in 1888, but this investigator has used the methylene blue stain. Dogiel, whose experiments are distinguished by skill and thoroughness, errs, however, in interpreting this finding. He definitely saw the stout varicose arborizations exhibited by the centrifugal fibers at the level of the spongioblasts, but he does not agree with me that the individual end-branches of these processes terminate freely and pericellularly, i.e. in the vicinity of or amongst the amacrine cells. Instead he believes that the branches of these fibers fuse with the protoplasmic processes of certain spongioblasts. According to this

(Continued on next page)

(Continued from preceding page)

assumption we would be dealing with a very special class of nervous elements in the retina: one whose protoplasmic branches converge to form an axis cylinder which then continues into an optic fiber. Such a discovery would be quite unusual and hitherto unknown, for no modern observer (such as Golgi, Cajal, Tartuferi, Retzius, van Gehuchten, von Lenhossèk, L. Sala, C. Caleja, P. Ramón, et al.) has found anything like this in the nervous system of either vertebrates or invertebrates.

It is remarkable that Dogiel should hold such a peculiar opinion purely on the basis of preparations and sections stained with methlyene blue, without feeling the need to employ another more modern staining method as a control. Certainly it was known to Dogiel that I had described the branches of the centrifugal fibers as terminating completely freely and that I based this conclusion on many entirely and absolutely clear sections which had been impregnated with chromium-silver. For this reason, rather than simply stating that I had made an error, Dogiel should have mentioned—if only once—the method which led me to my conclusions and to which we principally owe the discovery of the centrifugal fibers and their terminal ramifications. I am convinced that this Russian scholar might then have at least spoken in a less definitive tone about the problem at hand.

I repeat that, *because of the incomplete transparency of sections stained with methylene blue it is very difficult to study the finer relationships of cells to one another.* Branches which simply cross are too easily mistaken for the appearance of a net, i.e., a fusion of the cell processes with one another.

In the past several months I have tried to clarify this situation, employing both the chromium-silver and the methylene blue stains, and today I must confirm in its entirety my description of the centrifugal fibers made previously. Furthermore after following Dogiel's procedure with the methylene blue stain precisely, I could also convince myself that the terminal ramifications of the centrifugal fibers end completely freely.

On sections in which the centrifugal fibers are stained very deeply with methylene blue (retinae of pigeons, domestic fowl, house sparrows, etc.) the spongioblasts are usually quite incompletely stained or totally devoid of stain. If the terminal arborizations are examined with a powerful objective (Zeiss apochromat 1.30 or 1.40), it is very easy to determine that they terminate completely independently of one another. Sometimes it is possible to see that a nest does surround the cell body or the processes of the spongioblasts, but it is never possible to discover a trace of true fusion between both elements. Dogiel had mistaken a simple contact for a direct fusion. As can be seen from his figures, however, he at least grants that sometimes the varicose branches of the fibers appear beautifully and completely stained, whereas the spongioblasts and hence their alleged connecting branches remain unstained. This circumstance can be seen in his drawings, and in fact it alone speaks against Dogiel's conclusion.

So as not to neglect any control procedure, I have recently made sections through the retinae of pigeons and sparrows. In this series I saw more than 150 well stained centrifugal fibers with very varicose, thick end-branches surrounding the spongioblasts, as I described earlier. Sometimes the end-branches form a complete nest around the spongioblasts, which is reminiscent of the bed of nerve

EPITHELIAL CELLS

In Plate VI, Figure 4, I have drawn two epithelial cells from the retina of the chicken. It can be seen that they are very similar to those of the reptile and differ only in their delicacy and greater number of filaments in their descending clusters. Also the filaments are virtually smooth at the level of the inner plexiform zone. Only tiny outgrowths or spines can be seen on them. At the ganglion cell level these spines become twisted and increase somewhat in thickness. With the exception of the amacrine cells, which are quite incompletely protected, all of the elements of the nuclear layers are completely surrounded by the epithelial cells.*

REFERENCES

1. Ramón y Cajal, S.: Sur la morphologie et les connexions des éléments de la rétine des oiseaux. *Anat. Anz.*, 1889 (4), 111-121.
2. Schultze, M.: Über Stäbchen und Zapfen in der Retina. *Arch. f. mikrosk. Anat.*, 1867 (3). 215-247.
3. Schwalbe, G.: Mikroskopische Anatomie des Sehnerven, der Netzhaut, und des Glaskörpers. In von Graefe, A. and Saemisch, T. *Handbuch der gesammten Augenheilkunde*. Vol. 1, Leipzig, 1874, pp. .321-479.
4. Krause, W.: Die Membrana fenestrata der Retina. *Arch. f. Anat. u. Physiol.*, 1871.
5. Dobrowsky, W.: Zur Anatomie der Retina. *Arch. f. Anat., Physiol., u. wissensch. Med.*, 1871, p. 221.
6. Hoffmann, C.: Zur Anatomie der Retina. II. Über den Bau der Retina bei den Vögeln. *Niederl. Arch. f. Zool.*, 1877 (3), 217.

---

fibers which surrounds the body of the Purkinje cells in the cerebellum. Sometimes the final twigs ascend for a long stretch into the inner nuclear layer, but they never cross the upper border of the spongioblast zone. The fact that sometimes twigs are found which run backwards in the nuclear layer is significant, as it does not support Dogiel's viewpoint. One never finds a stained spongioblast—neither with chromium-silver nor with methylene blue—whose processes branch amongst the nuclei or which run backwards in any way or for any distance in the inner nuclear layer. Each process of a spongioblast descends immediately to reach the inner plexiform layer within which it forms its terminal arborization. (1894 edition)

* These cells have a large number of lateral facets and indentations in which the individual nuclei lie well-isolated, as though in a private box. (1894 edition)

7. Beauregard, M.: Contribution a l'étude du rouge rétinien. *J. d. l'Anat. et. d. la Physiol.*, 1879 (15), 161-174.
8. Schultze, M.: Über Stäbchen und Zapfen in der Retina. *Arch. f. mikrosk. Anat.*, 1867 (3), 215-247.
9. Hoffmann, C.: Zur Anatomie der Retina. III. Über den Bau der Retina bei den Vögeln. *Niederl. Arch. f. Zool.*, 1877 (3), 217.
10. Dogiel, A.: Zur Frage über den Bau der Nervenzellen und über das Verhältnis ihres Achsencylinders. *Arch. f. mikrosk. Anat.*, 1893 (41), 62-87.
11. von Monakow, C.: Experimentelle und pathologisch-anatomische Untersuchungen über die optischen Centren und Bahnen. *Arch. f. Psych.*, 1889 (20), 714-787.
12. Dogiel, A.: Zur Frage über den Bau der Nervenzellen und über das Verhältnis ihres Achsencylinder- (nerven-) Fortsatzes zu den protoplasmafortsätzen (Dendriten). *Arch. f. mikrosk. Anat.*, 1893 (41), 62-87.

Chapter VII

THE RETINA OF MAMMALS

THE mammalian retina is closely related to the retina of lower vertebrates. Even those modifications, which on first glance seem to be unique to man or mammals, can also be seen in nearly the same detail in nocturnal birds and bony fishes. Examples include the slenderness and extraordinary number of rods, the spherical shape of lower terminations of the rods which have no basilar fibers, the rather considerable thickness of the outer nuclear layer, etc.

I will not review the numerous studies which have been concerned with the mammalian retina. I would only like to point out the more recent ones: Schiefferdecker,[1] Borysiekiewicz,[2] Kuhnt,[3] Lenox,[4] Tartuferi,[5] Dogiel.[6] We should also not forget the classical collected works of Schwalbe[7] and Ranvier.[8] I myself published an earlier communication on the mammalian retina,[9] as well as a summary of this work in the *Manual de Histologia normal* (1889). Finally, two other earlier studies should also be mentioned: one by E. Baquis[10] and one by W. Krause.[11]

The important investigations of Tartuferi and Dogiel on the morphology of the retinal elements in mammals have been only partially replicated in the brief report of d'Ellia Baquis on the retina of the marten. It is, therefore, necessary at this point to submit the statements of these scholars to a controlled study. The two research techniques used by these investigators should be combined, so that the findings obtained with the methylene blue and chromium-silver stains can corroborate and enhance one another.

With this in mind, I set out to study successively the retina of the dog, cat, pig, mouse, sheep, horse, and ox. First it should be mentioned that the retinal structure of all these animals is virtually identical, so that the following description holds true for all these animals. The differences which I observed concern the relative thickness of the retinal layers and some variation in cell volume. The structure of every layer and the morphology of every type of cell, however, remains absolutely constant.

THE VISUAL CELL LAYER

My investigations can only confirm the classical descriptions. As Tartuferi noted, the chromium-silver technique stains the inner segments of the rods and cones more intensely than the outer segments.

THE LAYER OF VISUAL CELL NUCLEI

I have almost nothing to add to the descriptions of other authors, especially those of Tartuferi, who made his observations with the Golgi method. In my preparations the cone process is thick and virtually straight. The cone nucleus lies just below the outer limiting membrane, and the cone fiber terminates below in a conical swelling with fine basilar radiating fibers (Plate V, Fig. 2, *a*).

The rod fibers are very fine, twisted, and varicose. The rod nucleus may be situated at various levels between the outer limiting membrane and the outer plexiform layer. It is oval or polyhedral and surrounded by an extraordinarily thin layer of protoplasm.

The rod fibers end completely freely in a spherical or oval swelling at the outermost level of the outer plexiform layer. This situation occurs in all animals having thin rods and a thick outer nuclear layer (Plate V, Fig. 2, *b*).

The free ending of the granule or the lower footpiece of the rod often appears clearly on sections stained with carmine or hematoxylin. Indeed, in his studies of the retina, M. Schultze[12] correctly represented them as independent and freely-ending spherules. Unfortunately the prevailing bias, which held that the visual cells were continuous with the optic nerve fibers prevented this distinguished anatomist from describing something which he correctly observed and sketched. This is an eloquent example of the undesirable influence a preconceived notion can exert on even the best observers.

This influence can also be observed in the work of other

The Retina of Mammals

equally distinguished histologists, e.g. Tartuferi and Baquis. The methods used by these investigators would have permitted them to answer this question definitively. In the plate accompanying Tartuferi's work, rods can be seen which terminate below with free spherules; however, several others are found which are connected with the outer plexiform layer by means of very delicate fibers. Nevertheless, in the text describing the figures, Tartuferi completely disregards something which was so beautifully demonstrated to him and maintains that "the rod fiber terminates on the outer surface of the outer reticular layer; where it connects with a fiber of the subepithelial net, a varicosity is often seen."[5] From this passage it can be seen that Tartuferi regards the terminal spherule simply as a varicosity of a fiber which anastomoses with the net of the outer reticular layer. At least this follows from a consideration of the plate which he cited.

In my first study of the retina,[13] I demonstrated that this hypothesis is not tenable. In describing the rods of nocturnal birds I said: "In nocturnal birds, the rods are very thin and terminate freely below in the form of a very small round knob, just as do the rods of mammals." In my latest publication on the mammalian retina I energetically defended this doctrine, whose importance for the general theory of the connection of nervous elements is undeniable. Since then I have examined more than two-hundred successful preparations of the retina of the dog, pig, ox, etc., and I am even more convinced of my original opinion.

In his work on the human retina Dogiel[14] seems to have a favorable opinion of this hypothesis, for he says: "Although I have carefully examined a great number of preparations with very complete staining of the nervous elements of the retina, I have never been able to observe a direct connection between the feet of the neuroepithelial cells and the processes of the cellular elements of the Ganglia retinae." In the plates accompanying the text Dogiel also draws the terminal spherules of the rods as ending completely freely. However, in his most recent work,[15] he seems to be less convinced of this fact, because he claims to have seen one or two very fine, tiny fibers arising from these swellings and joining with the outer plexiform layer which lies beneath.

CONNECTION OF THE RODS AND CONES

The outer plexiform layer in mammals is divided into two distinct concentric strata: the outer stratum, or the layer containing the end-feet of the visual cells; and the inner stratum, or the layer containing the horizontal fibers.

A. The Outer Stratum

This is a poorly delimited zone whose granular appearance has been noted previously by other histologists. It is formed by the articulation of two types of fibers: The fibers and terminal spherules of the rods on the one hand, and the fine ascending terminal clusters of certain bipolar cells on the other (the bipolar cells destined for the rods). The connection between these two types of elements occurs in such a way that the rod spherules lie in the nooks formed by the fibers of the bipolar cell clusters (Plate V, Fig. 2, c).

Sometimes the terminal knobs of the rods may be seen to descend to the second stratum of the outer plexiform layer, where they make contact with the thick branches of the terminal clusters of the bipolar cells destined for the cones,* and perhaps also with the processes of the horizontal cells. However, this occurs very rarely and is difficult to observe.

B. The Inner Stratum

This layer is composed mainly of two levels: The upper level contains the pedicles or terminal swellings of the cones, whose laterally radiating fibers form a tight, thin horizontal plexus. The lower level is composed of a horizontal plexus with very fine branches, the majority of which arise from the flat extensions of the upper terminal clusters of those bipolar cells which

---

* Both the 1892 and 1933 French editions read "bipolares destinées aux bâtonnets" (bipolars destined for the rods), whereas the bold type of the 1894 German edition makes it very clear that the bipolars destined for the cones are involved: "bipolare Zellen, welche zu den *Zapfen* gehören."

I have called bipolar cells destined for the cones, so as to distinguish them from other types. The connection here is made only by contact, since the basilar filaments of the cones always end freely, just as do the terminal extensions of the bipolars.

The row formed in the second stratum of the outer plexiform layer by the terminal swellings of the cones is interrupted from time to time, so as to allow the ascending terminal clusters of the bipolar cells destined for the rods to pass through. Sometimes ascending terminal fibers can also be seen here which intermingle in both strata. These fibers arise either from the protoplasmic processes of the underlying horizontal cells or from the terminal ramifications of certain axis cylinders.

Outer Horizontal Cells (Outer Basilar Cells)

In the ox retina I have sometimes encountered small oval cells (Plate V, Fig. 4, *h*) with horizontal branches extending from their lower surface. They extend into the outer stratum of the outer plexiform layer, where they spread out and ramify. I never could establish the existence of a descending process, perhaps only because of incomplete impregnation of the preparation; hence I cannot say whether these cells correspond to the displaced bipolar cells which Dogiel has found in mammals (his subepithelial cells) or whether they are simply a special variety of horizontal or subreticular cell. Now and then ascending spines may be seen to arise from the processes of these cells as they extend horizontally. These spines project upward among the terminal knobs of the rods and always end with a small nodule.

HORIZONTAL CELL LAYER

Horizontal cells (basal cells, stellate cells, or subreticular cells of other workers) have been observed in the mammalian retina for some time: in the calf by Merkel[16] and Kölliker,[17] in the horse (where they appear to be especially well-developed) by Golgi and Manfredi[18] and by Rivolta,[19] in man by Schwalbe[20] and Dogiel,[21] in the cat by Ranvier,[22] and in a large number of other vertebrates by W. Krause[23] and by Schiefferdecker.[24]

The opinion of these investigators concerning the nature of

the horizontal cells varies considerably. In general, though, they are viewed as a type of stellate structural cell whose processes associate to form a concentric and continuous network. In contrast there are some authors, Rivolta for example, who prefer to regard them as nerve cells.

Similarly there is also a diversity of opinions concerning the different subtypes of these cells. According to Schiefferdecker there are two types of horizontal cell in mammalian retina: the intermediate concentric cells (my outer horizontal cells) and the inner concentric cells (probably my inner horizontal cells). The outer concentric cells (my displaced bipolar cells) are not present in mammals.

Tartuferi has also distinguished two types of horizontal cells: (a) the stellate or middle-sized cells ("cellule stellato" or "cellule superficiali di grandezza media"), which lie transversely in the outermost part of the inner nuclear layer, (b) the large superficial cells ("grosse cellule superficiali"), which are situated below the first type. They are characterized by the thickness of their horizontal protoplasmic branches, a few of which descend and disappear in the inner plexiform layer. In addition, these cells are especially distinguished by the presence of a branch which runs horizontally and exhibits all the characteristics of an axis cylinder.

Both of the cell types described by Tartuferi represent only one class according to Dogiel (large and small stellate cells). They differ only in size and not by their characteristics, which are exactly the same in both the large and the small stellate cells. Indeed, according to Dogiel, both of these types of cell have descending protoplasmic processes which branch in the inner plexiform layer. Furthermore, both cell types have an axis cylinder which travels first horizontally and then vertically, and eventually becomes an optic nerve fiber. Both are characterized ultimately by the fact that the horizontal processes which are distributed in the outer plexiform layer end as terminal clusters with short, varicose fibers of granulated appearance.

On the basis of a very thorough study of these horizontal cells in the mammal with the methods of both Dogiel and Golgi, I have arrived at the conviction that this Russian scholar found and described only *one* type of stellate or horizontal cell in the human retina. This cell type probably corresponds with the "grosse cellule superficiali" which Tartuferi described. The smaller type of horizontal cell (Tartuferi's "cellule superficiali di grandezza media" or "cellule stellato") is absent in both Dogiel's text and figures. This oversight is the more surprising, since these cells are very easily stained with methylene blue, showing no descending protoplasmic processes and having a very characteristic shape (Plate VII, Fig. 9).

In fact, two types of horizontal cells can be easily distinguished in the retina of all mammals (dog, cat, rabbit, pig, sheep, ox, etc.): the outer horizontal cells, which are very flat and distribute themselves exclusively in the outer plexiform layer; and the inner horizontal cells, which lie below and are significantly larger. This second type of cell may be further subdivided into cells with and without descending protoplasmic expansions.

Outer Horizontal Cells

These are very flat stellate elements which, as Tartuferi has already noted, lie in the outermost part of the inner nuclear layer and extend almost to the middle of the outer plexiform layer (Tartuferi's "cellule superficiali di grandezza media") (Plate V, Fig. 3, A and Plate VII, Fig. 7 and Fig. 10). Two varieties can be distinguished on the basis of size, although intermediate sizes are not absent: (a) small cells varying in diameter from 12μ-20μ which barely extend to the bipolar cell layer, and (b) quite voluminous cells which are sometimes as big as 40μ. This second type of cell has a conical or semilunar shape, the cell body being embedded in the outer plexiform layer.

If either the larger or smaller of these two cell types is examined in a horizontal section through the retina, a remarkably large number of diverging varicose, horizontal protoplasmic processes are seen which often ramify repeatedly. The terminal branches are very delicate and virtually straight. After taking a course which may be of considerable length, they end freely. These endings do not give off the terminal clusters of finger-like fibers, which are so characteristic of the processes of the inner horizontal cells. The outer horizontal cells often have another peculiarity, namely that their main branches show triangular swellings where they divide into two sub-branches.

Chromium-silver stains the protoplasmic processes a more or less pale coffee brown color, which seems to be caused by the vertical flattening which these expansions have undergone. Methylene blue stains them less intensely.

If all the cells in a certain area of the outer plexiform layer are stained, then it is possible to see that these cells are very numerous, and also that their diverging branches interlace tightly in all directions, thus forming a flat, very compact, and rich plexus (Plate VII, Fig. 9). At certain locations there are roundish spaces within this latticework. These spaces allow passage for the terminal clusters of the bipolars destined for the rods and for the end-feet of the cones.

In horizontal sections through the retina it is very difficult to determine the shape of the protoplasmic arborizations of the outer horizontal cells. It is possible, however, to observe nicely that tiny ascending spines often arise from the upper surface of the diverging branches and extend to the level of the visual cell end-feet.

The axis cylinder is very difficult to find because of the extremely numerous and delicate secondary and tertiary protoplasmic branches. This explains why Tartuferi was not able to see them. I myself have searched for them in vain for quite a long time. Nevertheless, if one closely examines horizontal sections with well-stained cells, a fine horizontal process can be seen. It usually arises along the course of a thick transverse protoplasmic process. This is the nerve process which I first discovered in the bird. After a horizontal and usually tortuous course, this axis cylinder ends with a few fine varicose branches in the outermost stratum of the outer plexiform layer. During its course it sends off collateral branches at a right angle; these in turn ramify repeatedly and terminate freely within this layer. The collateral branches and their terminal ramifications do not stain with methylene blue. I, at least, have never been able to stain them sufficiently well with methylene blue to study them (Plate VII, Fig. 7).

Inner Horizontal Cells

These cells (Tartuferi's "grosse cellule superficiali" and Dogiel's "grosse und kleine sternförmige Zellen") can be broken down into two types: horizontal cells with descending protoplasmic processes, and horizontal cells without such processes.

1. The Inner Horizontal Cells with Descending Processes

These cells have been well described by Tartuferi, Baquis, and especially by Dogiel. They are large cells of conical or pyramidal shape, with an inverted base; a number of thick horizontal processes are given off from them. These processes have the attribute noted by Tartuferi, i.e. that they taper off continuously and very rapidly, independently of the divisions which they produce (Plate VI, Fig. 13 and Fig. 12). These protoplasmic branches are in general much shorter than those of the outer horizontal cells, and after a few dichotomous divisions, it is typical for them to break up into clusters with short, gnarled, finger-like fibers which in turn terminate with small swellings (Plate VI, Fig. 13 and Fig. 14, *a;* also Plate VII, Fig. 6, *c*).

There is usually one very thick descending protoplasmic process which arises from the lower apex of the protoplasmic cell body and extends to the outer half of the inner plexiform layer. There it usually divides into two branches which extend more or less horizontally but in opposing directions. These branches, which usually occupy the second sublayer of the inner plexiform layer, sometimes redivide two or three times, thereby forming a very rich horizontal plexus. In other cases, however, they terminate without ever dividing, but only become gradually thinner and more delicate until they end completely (Plate VI, Fig. 12, *a* and Fig. 14). Now and then, instead of one descending protoplasmic branch, *two* descending protoplasmic processes can be seen (Plate VII, Fig. 6, *a, b*). These branches separate from one another at an acute angle, but terminate in the same way as the bifurcated branches which arise from a single trunk.

The axis cylinder is very thick. It begins with a conical swelling and courses horizontally, somewhat removed from the outer plexiform layer, over an enormous extent. Sometimes I have followed such a fiber for more than 0.8 mm without finding its termination. It has no collateral branches and never changes its direction. I also cannot agree with Dogiel, who claims to have seen the axis cylinder extending downward, ultimately to become a fiber of the optic nerve layer. I would much rather assume that this axis cylinder terminates in the outer plexiform layer itself by means of a free terminal arborization of enormous extent (Plate VII, Fig. 5, A). I will return to this very important point later.

2. The Inner Horizontal Cells with No Descending Processes

Judging from the descriptions of Tartuferi and Dogiel, neither investigator has seen this type of cell. Perhaps they assumed that the descending fibers of these cells simply were not stainable. At first I, too, was under the same impression, but after completing a number of studies with the staining methods of Golgi and of Dogiel, I have become convinced that in fact the majority of inner horizontal cells have no vertical processes. The lower aspect of the cell body appears quite rounded, and there is no suggestion of a broken or incompletely stained process (Plate VI, Fig. 12, b and Plate VII, Fig. 5).

Two types of these elements can be distinguished: (a) fusiform or semilunar cells with very few protoplasmic processes arising from their lower surface; these processes course horizontally (Plate VII, Fig. 5, A, C), and (b) very large cells with a very protuberant lower surface; these cells have a large number of diverging processes (Plate VI, Fig. 13 and Fig. 12, b).

The nerve process is very thick and often takes its origin from a protoplasmic branch. It extends horizontally rather considerably at some distance from the outer plexiform layer. Sometimes the process bows a bit downward before it continues its horizontal course.

Nerve Fibers which Branch in the Outer Plexiform Layer

When this layer is well stained, three types of nerve endings can be differentiated in a horizontal section: thick fibers, running parallel to the retinal surface, which have flat arborizations of considerable extent; somewhat thinner fibers which run horizontally and break up into less profuse ramifications; and abundant collateral fibers which arise from a branch that ascends from within the inner plexiform layer.

1. Thick Fibers with Extensive Terminal Ramifications

This is the most important fact which my latest investigations with the Golgi method have revealed to me in the mammalian retina (cat, dog, ox, etc.).

When a section parallel to the retinal surface is examined, especially if the retina has been converted to a thick block by the rolling-up method, a large number of thick horizontal axis cylinders can be seen crossing one another in every possible direction in the outermost portion of the inner nuclear layer, i.e. below the outer plexiform layer. These fibers divide dichotomously several times, and their branches gradually extend more sclerally as they approach their termination. As soon as the branches or their ramifications have reached the deep part of the outer plexiform layer (the second stratum), they become noticeably thicker and quite varicose; ultimately they dissolve into a flat, rich terminal arborization. This arborization has twisted, moniliform and diverging branches which extend over an enormously wide area in that layer (Plate VI, Fig. 7). Small ascending spines can be seen arising from the contours of the secondary and tertiary branches. These spines extend among the rod spherules, i.e. they terminate in the outer stratum of the outer plexiform layer with a roundish swelling.

If the impregnation of the retina is very complete, the lower stratum of the outer plexiform layer in a horizontal section is literally completely filled with a very large number of these ramifications which in turn are mixed with the protoplasmic expansions of the outer horizontal cells, thereby forming a remarkably rich and complicated lattice.

In perpendicular sections the primary and secondary ramifications appear only in cross section, and it is difficult to follow them. In contrast their projecting, ascending collaterals or spines are seen very nicely, and extend to the stratum of the terminal knobs of the visual cells (Plate VI, Fig. 10). Small polygonal spaces can be seen between the secondary and tertiary branches which appear to be occupied by the cone pedicles (Plate VI, Fig. 8, *a*.)

2. Fibers with Less Extensive End-branches

In addition to the thick fibers which have such enormous ramifications, other somewhat thinner fibers can be found. These occupy the same stratum and are oriented in the same direction; their terminal ramifications are less extensive, but otherwise have the same characteristics which were just described above (Plate VI, Fig. 8).

Both types of terminal arborizations occur in all mammals (ox, dog, cat, rabbit, etc.), but it seems to me that their extent is proportional to the size of the retina. Thus, in a young rabbit (15 days old) they appear rather small and very varicose (Plate VI, Fig. 9), whereas in the ox they extend over a remarkably large area (Plate VI, Fig. 7).

What is the origin of these arborizing fibers? I believe that they must be regarded as the axis cylinders of the large, inner horizontal cells (cells with no descending processes, and also cells which do have such descending processes). The relatively thin fibers probably represent the axis cylinders of the smaller horizontal cells, whereas the thicker fibers would represent the continuation of the nerve processes of the larger, inner horizontal cells.

The reasons which have led me to this particular conclusion are the following:

1. In one case I succeeded in directly identifying the continuity between such fibers and the axis cylinder of an inner horizontal cell without a descending process (Plate VII, Fig. 5, *B*).

2. The branched fibers never descend below the level of the horizontal cell layer. This has been observed in approximately one hundred sections in which the axis cylinders have been demonstrated to be quite adequately stained. This negative finding is important. It is thus not possible for me to concur with Dogiel's opinion that the axis cylinders of the inner horizontal cells descend vertically, after taking a brief horizontal course, in order then to become fibers of the optic nerve fiber layer. Moreover, the same results are obtained with methylene blue as with

chromium-silver with regard to this particular point. The ramified fibers are never seen to change their character (level of arborization), although they can be followed over a wide area. Incidentally, it has been observed that methylene blue very often stains the main branches of the arborization, but it is not capable of revealing the very characteristic secondary and tertiary branches.

3. The axis cylinder of the inner horizontal cells is just about as thick as the large ramified fibers. Furthermore, the position and direction of the two types of fibers is identical.

3. Fine Fibers Arising from the Inner Plexiform Layer

Sometimes in preparations which have been treated with the double impregnation method, certain delicate fibers which proceed from the inner plexiform layer can be seen. These ascend vertically to the outer plexiform layer where they break up into a ramification with very gnarled, horizontal branches (Plate V, Fig. 2, *i*). These peculiar terminal fibers can also be found in the frog and teleost fish. In some cases it can be established that these fibers take a horizontal course at the level of the inner plexiform layer, so that it is impossible to pursue these fibers completely, and thus to discover their origin.

Before we leave the horizontal cell layer, I must mention yet another group of cells. These have already been noted by d'Ellia Baquis under the name of the communicating pyramidal cells ("cellule piramidali comunicanti"). These are very large pyramidal cells. They are inverted so that the base of the pyramid lies more externally than the apex, which impinges on the inner plexiform layer below. Numerous processes arise from their upper surface, and these extend to the outer plexiform layer. Their apex elongates into a thick branch which is lost at the level of the first sublayer of the inner plexiform layer. Since I have not detected these peculiar cells in many species of mammals which I have examined, I believe that we are dealing with a morphological modification of some cells, which Tartuferi, Dogiel, or I myself have already described. It would be possible that the aforesaid pyramidal cells are simply inner horizontal cells with a descending process (Tartuferi's "grosse cellule superficielli") whose axis cylinder has not been stained for some reason. Perhaps the shape and the descending terminal cluster of these cells is somewhat modified in the marten.

BIPOLAR CELL LAYER

General Information on the Bipolar Cells

My own investigations completely support those of Tartuferi and Dogiel, especially as regards the general morphology of the bipolar cells.

The bipolar cell bodies of mammals are much bigger and more irregularly-shaped than those of lower vertebrates, but they too have two processes, an ascending and a descending one.

The ascending process is frequently multiple. It is very thick and forms a very profuse arborization at the level of the outer plexiform layer. The descending process descends in a nearly straight line, crosses the amacrine cell layer, and terminates at varying levels in the inner plexiform layer with a short and very varicose arborization.

As in all vertebrates, the terminal branches of both the upper and the lower clusters always end completely freely with more or less thick swellings. This fact is so easy to establish, particularly in the lower terminal clusters of the bipolar cells, that were it not for the unfortunate influence of prejudice, it would be indeed difficult to understand how two such careful observers as Tartuferi and Dogiel could describe a net of anastomoses between the clusters of neighboring cells.

Dogiel describes a type of fiber in the upper terminal clusters which exhibits all the characteristics of a Landolt club. I have not been able to find such fibers in my own preparations, although in the last few months I have often searched for them in dog, sheep, and ox retinae stained with methylene blue. I have also never succeeded in impregnating such a fiber with the Golgi method, even when the double or triple impregnation procedure was used. This situation is indeed odd, in view of the fact that the Landolt clubs of frogs, reptiles, and birds can be stained very reliably with chromium-silver.

The Different Types of Bipolar Cells

If the bipolar cells of mammals are carefully compared with one another, differences can soon be noted, especially with regard to the level and form of the ascending cluster. These differences, in combination with the other physiological characteristics which reliably distinguish bipolar cells, allow three classifications of cell types: bipolar cells with vertically ramifying clusters, or bipolars destined for the rods; bipolar cells with flat ramifying clusters, or bipolars destined for the cones; giant bipolar cells with very extensive upper clusters.

1. Bipolar Cells with an Ascending Cluster

Tartuferi described just this one type of bipolar cell. Judging from his drawings, the branches of the upper cluster always extend upward and become gradually thinner. Moreover, this is readily understood since these very cells are stained easily and regularly with the Golgi method. On the other hand, it appears that Dogiel succeeded in staining only the bipolars destined for the cones, because all of the cells of this type which he sketched show an upper cluster which spreads horizontally with very sparse terminal fibers. Furthermore, the term which Dogiel chose for these processes which extend to the outer plexiform layer ("horizontale Fortsätze") also supports this idea.*

The bipolar cells with vertically ascending clusters, which are destined for the rods (Plate V, Fig. 2) are thick and oval or semilunar. They have a variable number of branches which divide at acute angles and then continue as collateral branches. These divide in turn and ascend to the upper stratum of the outer plexiform layer where they end freely at different levels. The final ending is sharp and often has at its end an extremely delicate varicosity.

The angles formed by the secondary and tertiary branches are usually rounded, so that the space between the ascending fibers conforms in size and shape to that of the rod spherules.

---

* Like chromium-silver, methylene blue preferentially stains one variety of bipolar cell: the bipolar cells with horizontal clusters destined for the cones are seen almost exclusively. (1892 edition)

As we have said previously, this interspace serves for the insertion of the rod spherules with which nervous contact is made. By means of these connections the bipolar cell receives the activity from many rods. Moreover this relationship can be observed directly in certain preparations where the chromium-silver has simultaneously impregnated both parts of this neural articulation (Plate V, Fig. 2, c and Fig. 4, a).

The descending fiber is very long and traverses the entire inner plexiform layer. Directly over the upper surface of the ganglion cells (Fig. 2, n), it breaks up into a short arborization with thick, moniliform branches whose terminations exhibit round or oval swellings. In some cases it seems to me as if a terminal arborization is formed in one of the sublayers of the inner plexiform layer. Finally, one sometimes sees a terminal ramification which is so simply constructed that it consists only of one bifurcation with short diverging branches ending in terminal knobs.

The relative dimensions of the ascending cluster are quite variable. In this respect the bipolars destined for the rods can be subdivided into giant and small cells, although there are also transitional forms between these two main types. The larger cells have an upper cluster with such profuse ascending fibers that they make contact with fifteen to twenty rod spherules, whereas the smaller ones (Plate V, Fig. 2, d) possess only a very small number of ascending fibers so that they contact only three or four rod spherules.

2. Bipolar Cells with Horizontal Clusters Destined for the Cones

These occur at every level of the bipolar cell layer, but they are most abundant in the neighborhood of the amacrine cells. The upper cluster reaches the deep stratum of the outer plexiform layer and extends laterally over a much wider area than the ascending clusters of the bipolars destined for the rods (Plate V, Fig. 2, e and Fig. 4, b, c, d, e). The terminal branches, which are very fine and long, never have ascending spines. They end completely freely after interlacing many times with the branches of neighboring bipolar cells. The plexus thus formed has branches which spread laterally just below the end-feet of the cones, so that they probably contact the cone pedicles and terminal fibers. The fibers of the bipolar cells in question never reach the outer stratum of the outer plexiform layer where the terminal spherules of the rods are located. Conversely, the rod spherules never, or only very seldom, descend to the second stratum of the outer plexiform layer, i.e. to the region of the cone end-feet.

Just as in the teleost fish, two distinct pathways for the two types of light stimulus are found in the mammal. One is dominated by the cones, and the other, by the rods. However, I do not believe that these two paths are completely isolated. I assume only that one type of light sensation is predominantly conducted in each pathway. Given the present observations, it is impossible to assume that the few rod spherules which do descend to the deeper stratum of the outer plexiform layer do not make additional contact with the terminal clusters of the bipolar cells destined for the cones but rather make exclusive contact with the lowest branches of the bipolar cells for the rods.* The descending process extends to the inner plexiform layer, where it forms a flat and rather varicose ramification that is often finer than that of the bipolars with an ascending terminal cluster (Plate V, Fig. 4). These terminal arborizations are arranged in five levels of successively deeper plexuses whose position coincides with the sublayers of the inner plexiform layer. The arborizations which lie in the fifth sublayer probably also touch the upper surface of certain ganglion cells, although this is quite rare. Sometimes, in addition to the terminal cluster a few collateral branches can be seen which ramify in a more superficial sublayer; this particular arrangement, however, is the exception for the mammals, whereas it is the general rule for the frog, reptile, and bird.

The fact that the descending cluster of the bipolar cells occupies different levels of the inner plexiform layer in mammals

---

* I am now in agreement with this last opinion, because I am persuaded that the rod spherules do make contact with the indentations of the bipolar cells destined for these receptor elements. Sometimes this contact is very intimate. (1933 edition)

has already been noted by Dogiel in the human retina. This finding is most significant if it is considered along with another fact which my research has revealed in all five classes of vertebrates: Each one of these sublayers of the inner plexiform layer is the exclusive region of ramification of a single-layered ganglion cell. These ganglion cells might well receive the impulses transmitted to them from the bipolars destined for the cones and conduct them, perfectly isolated, to optic centers. A similar connection might be established at a different level of the inner plexiform layer between the terminal clusters of the bipolars destined for the rods and single-layered ganglion cells. It is easy to understand that if the hypothesis of Tartuferi and Dogiel of a continuous net at each of the different sublayers of the inner plexiform layer is accepted, then individual transmission of the diverse elements forming the retinal image (points, lines differently colored or differently illuminated surfaces) could not be assumed.*

3. Giant Bipolar Cells

Although these cells could be included in the category of bipolar cells destined for the cones, I prefer to describe them separately. They are large, conical, or pyramidal cells which lie directly below the outer plexiform layer (Plate V, Fig. 2, *f* and Fig. 4, *g*). Many diverging processes arise from their upper surface and branch repeatedly, extending horizontally over a considerable distance. The plexus formed by these ramifications appears to lie in the second stratum of the outer plexiform layer. The arborization usually has an enormous lateral extent, as can be seen in Plate V, Figure 2, *f*. It seems to come into contact preferentially with the cone pedicles. However, in individual cases (Plate V, Fig. 4, *f*, *g*) tiny ascending spines can be seen which appear to turn toward the first stratum, i.e. the stratum of the rod spherules.

The descending process behaves just like that of other bipolar

---

* How can the isolated transmission and perception of a single sensation, such as a point, be explained if there were so many nerve net associations among the retinal cells? (1894 edition)

cells, so that at the level of the inner plexiform layer it forms a flat arborization which is very varicose and gnarled. All ramifications of these cells so far observed appear to lie in the fifth sublayer; however, the cell shown in Plate V, Figure 4, *f* does send one branch to the third sublayer.

The giant bipolar cells were apparently not stained by either Tartuferi or Dogiel. In one of Dogiel's illustrations, though, I find a cell which he described in the text as a stellate cell (my inner horizontal cells). Its properties are similar to those of the giant bipolar cells, but it has a descending cluster which is very small and varicose.

AMACRINE CELL LAYER

General Information

In his frequently cited work Tartuferi described several types of amacrine cells or spongioblasts: (a) Spongioblasts with a relatively thick, short process which divides repeatedly, ultimately filling a large part of the inner plexiform layer with its ramifications. According to Tartuferi's sketches, these cells are probably the same as those which I termed "neuroglia-shaped spongioblasts" (diffuse amacrine cells) in the avian retina. (b) Spongioblasts with a trunk which first descends and then breaks up into a very small number of horizontal branches. These cells undoubtedly correspond to my pyriform spongioblasts with a straight trunk which forms a horizontal arborization. These are the most abundant form of amacrine cell. (c) Voluminous mitral spongioblasts whose cell body is elongated into two or more processes which extend over the outer part of the inner plexiform layer. These are probably the spongioblasts which ramify at the level of the first sublayer.

Tartuferi has classified the amacrine cell types by their morphological characteristics which, comparatively speaking, are not as important as other features, such as the form of the terminal arborization and the inner plexiform sublayer in which these cells arborize. Actually the shape of the cell and its terminal arborization depends on which sublayer of the inner plexiform layer the terminal arborization is located. Thus, the amacrine cells of the first sublayer, which have no need for a descending branch, are multipolar and rather flat, whereas with a few minor exceptions, the amacrine cells of the fourth and fifth sublayers all have a straight vertical trunk which arborizes exclusively within the level of the plexus to which they contribute.

It is very important that the pyriform amacrine cells form superposed concentric plexuses which meet with the plexuses of the ganglion cells and with the terminal clusters of the bipolar cells. I first established this in the avian retina, but at first found only two plexuses or fibrillar sublayers in the inner plexiform layer. In the course of my further studies in the frog and reptile retinae,[25] however, I came to distinguish three or four sublayers. These sublayers of the inner plexiform layer are formed mainly by the junction of (a) the clusters of the pyriform amacrine cells which have a long, straight, descending trunk; (b) the flattened arborizations of the ganglion cells; and (c) the lower terminal clusters of the bipolar cells. In my later work on the mammalian retina[26] I was able to establish a similar relation, although here the layers formed by the horizontal clusters of the pyriform amacrine cells were less clear than in the lower vertebrates.

Recently, in a work which appeared at almost the same time as my study on the mammalian retina, Dogiel[27] described two types of spongioblasts in the human retina: the nervous spongioblasts and the spongioblasts with no axis cylinder (my amacrine cells).

One notes with some surprise that Dogiel describes only those nonnervous spongioblasts which I have called diffuse or unstratified cells, although there are a few elements which can be classified as monostratified cells of the first sublayer. The long and admirable series of stratified spongioblasts with straight trunks which form concentric plexuses are absent from the Russian scholar's description. This is understandable, in view of the fact that methylene blue, which Dogiel used exclusively, stains hardly any of the stratified amacrine cells. Instead, this stain preferentially impregnates the diffuse amacrine cells, as can be seen in my Plate VII, Figure 8. In this figure I have represented amacrine cells as they appeared in my preparations done with the Ehrlich-Dogiel method.

Besides the spongioblasts mentioned above, Dogiel mentions cells which have the following peculiarity: The ramified processes which arise from the lower surface of the cell body form a very profuse plexus extending through a large part of the inner plexiform layer; axis cylinders are said to originate from the union of several fibrils in this plexus and ultimately to become optic nerve fibers. For my part, I could never establish this remarkable organization in any retina of any animal; I am convinced that Dogiel was led to this curious interpretation solely by the lack of clarity afforded by the methylene blue method, which is inadequate for displaying the finest terminal fibers of cells. But even if this mode of ending by a nerve fiber were to prove true, it would be an entirely isolated finding, because the investigations of Retzius[28] and Lenhossèk[29] have shown that even among the invertebrates—among which a similar hypothesis was made on the basis of better evidence—the axis cylinder always represents an extension of a single cell process.

According to Dogiel the nervous spongioblasts, i.e. those which send out an axis cylinder that is continuous with an optic nerve fiber, behave in a special way in the human retina. After the protoplasmic processes have divided several times, they are said to form a horizontal plexus lying sometimes in the outer, sometimes in the middle, and sometimes in the inner third of the inner plexiform layer. Thus, there are said to be three types of nerve cells in the amacrine cell layer, which can be distinguished by the level of the inner plexiform layer in which the protoplasmic processes ramify.

If Dogiel's sketches are carefully examined, it can be concluded that Dogiel has deceived himself, having most probably described certain nonnervous spongioblasts of the third, fourth, and fifth sublayers as actual nerve cells.

One need only compare the cells of my Plate V, Figure 7, C with Dogiel's Plate XXII, Figure 13, C to become convinced of how easy it is to make serious errors when the methylene blue method is employed. Both sketches evidently show the same type of spongioblast, but whereas hardly any processes can be seen in Dogiel's figure, a number of them can be discerned in mine. One of these processes extends to the neighborhood of the ganglion cells and might be mistaken for an axis cylinder, if it were incompletely stained. Luckily, in contrast to methylene blue, chromium-silver stains not only the descending process, which does resemble a nerve process in appearance, but also the exceptionally fine fibrils of its terminal cluster which lie within the level of the fifth sublayer. If the majority of the spongioblasts which Dogiel has stained with methylene blue are comparable to those which I stained with chromium-silver, then I come to the unavoidable conclusion that the chromium-silver stain shows very lovely terminal ramifications, including their finest processes, whereas the methylene blue stain shows only a few branches which are very difficult to study, especially as regards their termination.

The reservations which I have about the three types of nervous spongioblasts described by Dogiel in man are further justified by the fact that I have never seen an axis cylinder in these elements, despite countless preparations of the mammalian retina which I have made during the course of more than a year's work. With both staining methods the cell body and the protoplasmic extensions are quite well delineated. The mitral-shaped nervous spongioblasts (Dogiel's spongioblasts in the first third of the plexiform layer) are totally absent in my recent sections, so that I am now dubious about their existence in the mammal. Although I myself mentioned them in earlier work, it was at a time when I had not yet studied the amacrine cells of the fifth sublayer sufficiently (Plate V, Fig. 7, *C* and Plate VII, Fig. 8, *d*). In completely-stained preparations these cells are very similar to those having a true nerve process, which are found in the retinae of birds, reptiles, and frogs.

If it is assumed that the nervous spongioblasts are absent in mammals one might speculate on whether these cells have migrated from their usual location to the ganglion cell layer, where they might be represented by certain giant pyriform ganglion cells that arborize in the first sublayer. There is a circumstance which argues in favor of this interpretation. The latter type of cell is especially numerous in mammals, whereas in reptiles and birds, which have nervous spongioblasts, they are very rare. Indeed, a change in the position of a cell is not unheard of. Recall, for example, the displaced bipolars of the reptiles and frogs, which cannot be found in birds or teleost fishes.

From the physiological point of view, a change in the location of the retinal cells is without significance, provided that the level of protoplasmic arborizations and the direction of their functional processes remains constant, as is the case in the example at hand. Also, in displaced bipolar cells, both connecting organelles (processes destined for the outer plexiform layer and the lower terminal clusters) retain their normal position. In the displaced ganglion cells (nervous spongioblasts) there is no change in the organization of the protoplasmic clusters. Regardless of the position of the cell body these cells are distributed within the first sublayer of the inner plexiform layer.

In interpreting the nature of nerve cells, one should always consider the position and the connections of the protoplasmic and nerve processes to be of the greatest importance, more so than the location of the cell body itself. This is an important rule, a type of criterion, which can also be employed advantageously in other parts of the nervous system.

Special Description of the Amacrine Cells

In general these elements in mammals are similar to the amacrine cells of other vertebrates, i.e. in form, number, location, and arrangement of terminal arborizations, etc. However, in mammals the fibrils of the radical clusters and those of the gnarled arborizations do not attain the extraordinary length seen in the frog, reptile, and bird. There are five sublayers of arborization in the inner plexiform layer, though they are more difficult to differentiate than in other vertebrates. This is because of their considerable thickness and the lack of a precise planar distribution of the processes of several ganglion cells and the amacrine cells. The individual sublayers are less distinct also because the lower terminal clusters of the bipolar cells very often do not spread flatly.

A. Diffuse Amacrine Cells

Two varieties occur: the small cells and the large cells.

1. The Small Amacrine Cells

These cells have an oval or pyriform cell body from which there arises a descending process which soon breaks up into an arborization with very varicose diagonal branches that terminate in the lower two-thirds of the inner plexiform layer (Plate V, Fig. 8, *D*).

2. The Large Amacrine Cells

These cells have a triangular, semilunar, or mitral cell body. Two or three processes arising from their lower surface descend diagonally, divide repeatedly, and become quite varicose. Their terminal branches occupy almost the entire inner plexiform layer, although those branches which terminate as small swellings appear to accumulate preferentially in the fifth sublayer, directly above the ganglion cells (Plate V, Fig. 2, *h*).*

B. Stratified Amacrine Cells

1. The First Sublayer

As in the bird, these cells are semilunar or cuboidal, and they vary greatly in size. Several diverging branches arise from their lower surface and extend over a very wide area in the outermost part of the inner plexiform layer (Plate V, Fig. 7, *A*).

In addition to these cells, another less frequent variety is found. These are characterized by the extraordinary number and delicacy of their diverging processes, which divide only in the immediate area of the cell body. They course over a large expanse in the first and second sublayers, where they terminate freely (Plate V, Fig. 8, *A*).

---

* These cells stain very easily with methylene blue (Plate VII, Fig. 8, *f*). Often it is only these elements which will be stained. Moreover their descending branches can be seen to form a continuous, very granular zone within all of the fifth sublayer (Plate VII, Fig. 8, *g*). (1892 edition)

2. Amacrine Cells of the Second Sublayer

I have recognized three types of these cells: (a) very voluminous, pyriform cells with a thick trunk which breaks up at the level of the second sublayer into three or four stout horizontal branches of great length (Plate V, Fig. 7, *B*); (b) small pyriform cells whose descending trunk forms a magnificent radiation of straight, delicate, varicose branches which resemble nerve fibrils (Plate V, Fig. 8, *C*). (These are the amacrine cells with radial clusters which I described previously in the lower vertebrates.); (c) giant semilunar cells which are characterized by the fact that these give off two opposing branches which ramify within the second sublayer (Plate VI, Fig. 12, *c*). These cells are also often stained with methylene blue.

3. Amacrine Cells of the Third Sublayer

Here the same types of cells can be seen as in birds and reptiles: (a) giant cells with a few thick, horizontal processes which are given off from a stout vertical trunk and which have only scanty arborizations (Plate V, Fig. 8, *G*). (Their terminal branches are much shorter than in the reptile and they end freely with a large varicosity.); (b) small pyriform cells whose vertical trunk forms a lovely stellate radiation with very long, fine processes (Plate V, Fig. 7, *D*); (c) small cells, also pyriform, whose descending process breaks up into a very gnarled, sinuous ramification of moderate extent (Plate V, Fig. 8, *F* and Fig. 9, *B*, *C*).

4. Amacrine Cells of the Fourth Sublayer

Three different types of cells can be distinguished: (a) a type with a flat, radial cluster which is composed of very delicate long fibrils (Plate V, Fig. 8, *E*); (b) another type, also pyriform, whose terminal arborization is short, varicose, and very compact (Plate V, Fig. 7, *G*); (c) a giant type which is similar to that seen in the third sublayer with thick, horizontal terminal branches. Sometimes only two branches can be found, these projecting in opposite directions (Plate VI, Fig. 12).

5. Amacrine Cells of the Fifth Sublayer

Different cell types can also be recognized here: (a) a voluminous pyriform type, whose vertical trunk quickly divides into several thick branches. (These branches spread horizontally to form a sinuous and quite varicose ramification directly above the ganglion cells [Plate V, Fig. 7, *E*].); (b) a voluminous semilunar or tetragonal type, with fine branches projecting from its lower and lateral aspects. These branches give off many ramifications which reach the lower part of the fifth sublayer to form a fine, complicated, and very extensive plexus. In descending, a portion of these fibers goes first directly downward and then somewhat diagonally, so that during their course they traverse a large part of the inner plexiform layer. Finally a few of the processes which arise from the outer edges of the cell body appear to ramify in the first sublayer (Plate V, Fig. 7, *C*), so that these elements might be regarded as two-layered cells ("cellules bistratifées"). In addition, they have the property that methylene blue stains them intensely. Only in those sections treated with chromium-silver, however, can the extraordinary abundance and course of these very fine fibrils be seen completely.

6. Special Cells with an Ascending Axis Cylinder

Among the amacrine cells, I have observed two elements situated among the amacrine cells in the dog retina (Plate V, Fig. 2, *g*). They differ greatly from other cells of the inner nuclear layer. The cell body is triangular or oval in shape, and it has several descending processes projecting from the lower surface. These processes resemble protoplasmic processes and disappear in the upper half of the inner plexiform layer. There is also a fine process which arises from the upper surface of these cells which has the characteristics of an axis cylinder. It ascends, sometimes directly and sometimes obliquely, to the outer plexiform layer where it ends freely with a very short, varicose ramification.

In several hundred preparations I have observed only two cells of this type, so that I would not like to speculate about their significance.

7. Interstitial Amacrine Cells, or Amacrine Cells of the Inner Plexiform Layer

From Dogiel's work we are aware of displaced ganglion cells and displaced bipolar cells. These cells are found in a location other than that occupied by the majority of the same type of cells. In the mammalian retina displaced amacrine cells are also found scattered here and there in different sublayers of the inner plexiform layer (Plate V, Fig. 4, *i, j, m*). But although the cell body has moved to a different position, the processes of these cells still arborize in a horizontal plexus entirely in accordance with the rule for the arrangement of the amacrine cells.

The existence of such cells within the inner plexiform layer has already been noted by several workers, namely Nagel[30] and H. Müller.[31] More recently Borysiekiewicz[32] noted the presence of these cells in carnivores. He describes them as nerve cells with protoplasmic expansions, which could be subdivided into small and large types.

In the ox retina this type of cell is fusiform or triangular with a general orientation which is approximately parallel with that of the surface of the retina. Their expansions resemble those of the stratified amacrine cells, branching repeatedly and extending over a large horizontal area. Often after many divisions, the collaterals go to a different plexus or sublayer, such that each individual cell may provide terminal branches to two or three retinal plexuses. The terminal branches are very delicate and end freely.

The location of the displaced amacrine cells is quite variable. However most of these cells which I have seen in my own preparations are in the second sublayer, along with almost all their processes. Occasionally they occupy the third or even the fourth sublayer (Plate V, Fig. 4, *j, m*).

In addition to the horizontal amacrine cells, other triangular or irregularly-shaped amacrine cells with processes extending in a very variable direction can sometimes be found. For example, the cell shown in Plate VI, Figure 12, *K* gives rise to two types of processes: (a) ascending processes which send their ramifications to the second and first sublayers, and (b) more numerous descending processes which divide repeatedly and form a very complicated, varicose plexus in the fifth sublayer. Thus, we have an amacrine cell which belongs to two layers (bistratified amacrine cell).

Perhaps new staining attempts will reveal more cells of this type which occupy still other sublayers. It is also likely that displaced ganglion cells will be found, as in the reptile. This point, however, awaits further investigation.

GANGLION CELL LAYER
A. Single-layered Branched Ganglion Cells
1. The First Sublayer

Three main types are found here: (a) The giant type is a multipolar or bipolar cell which is semilunar or oval in shape. They give off very stout ascending branches from their upper surface, which upon arrival at the first sublayer, or at the space between the first and second sublayers, form a magnificent flat terminal ramification with thick branches that twist and divide extensively (Plate V, Fig. 9, *a*). (b) The small type of oval cells have a long ascending process which forms a delicate, wavy, horizontal ramification at the level of the first sublayer. Sometimes instead of a single ascending branch, two or more processes can be observed which disappear within the first sublayer after repeated divisions (Plate V, Fig. 7, *c*). (c) The last type of cell is middle-sized. I have noted them in the dog, particularly (Plate V, Fig. 9, *f* and Fig. 8, *f*). They are pyriform cells with a thick ascending trunk which gives off a highly developed varicose ramification in the first sublayer and in a portion of the second sublayer. Sometimes other types of cells are seen projecting to the same location. They are characterized by a very loose and more delicate ramification (Plate V, Fig. 9, *h*).

2. Ganglion Cells of the Second Sublayer

We have just seen that certain cells of the first sublayer extend their branches into the second sublayer; however, the second sublayer also contains special ramifications from other cells which can be placed in two categories:

(a) *The small variety.* These are pyriform cells with a delicate ascending branch which forms a thin arborization with long, slim filaments in the second sublayer (Plate V, Fig. 8, *a* and Plate VI, Fig. 12, *e*). Sometimes the terminal ramification is comprised solely of two horizontal branches which extend in opposite directions.

(b) *The giant variety.* These are semilunar or oval cells which often have a number of very thick ascending branches. The terminal fibers of these branches gather at the level of the second sublayer after multiple divisions and form a loose but very extensive plexus. The very thick and numerous, gnarled branches end freely (Plate V, Fig. 9, *c, e*). The remarkably large axis cylinder often arises from a protoplasmic branch. In several cases the giant ramifications of these ganglion cells are not confined exclusively to the second sublayer, but may also encroach upon the plexuses of the second and third sublayers.

3. Ganglion Cells of the Third Sublayer

(a) *The giant type.* These cells are pyriform and of rather considerable size. Their thick ascending trunk forms a sparse flat arborization with very stout branches at the level of the third sublayer (Plate V, Fig. 7, *e*).

(b) *The small type.* In the dog I have found a small multipolar cell whose ascending processes form a short, extremely varicose, and very dense arborization at the level of the third sublayer and in a portion of the fourth sublayer (Plate V, Fig. 8, *g*). The axis cylinder, which arises from a protoplasmic branch, descends to become a fiber of the optic nerve layer.

4. Ganglion Cells of the Fourth Sublayer

(a) *The small type.* These correspond to the quite remarkable small cells encountered in the lower vertebrates, especially in the bird and reptile. However, in the mammal the horizontal ramification is less profuse and not so compact. In the ox retina I found two varieties that can be easily distinguished from one another: pyriform cells with a very fine and varicose terminal cluster (Plate V, Fig. 7, *a*), and pyriform cells with a more extensive and loose terminal cluster (Plate V, Fig. 8, *e*).

(b) *The middle-sized type.* Pyriform or multipolar cells which are relatively large can be seen especially well in the dog retina. Their terminal ramification is extraordinarily rich and compact, and occupies all of the fourth sublayer and a good portion of the fifth sublayer (Plate V, Fig. 9, *g*, *d*). Perhaps this variety is simply a modification of the small type.

(c) *The type with a very extensive ramification.* In the ox retina I saw a rather large multipolar cell (Plate V, Fig. 7, *d*) with four or five ascending branches, each of which formed a cluster of very long fibers which coursed horizontally at the level of the fourth sublayer.

5. Ganglion Cells of the Fifth Sublayer

These cells stain very rarely, but I have been able to distinguish two types. Others will probably be found in further staining attempts, because this sublayer is quite thick and very rich in protoplasmic branches.

(a) *The large type with relatively thick branches* (Plate V, Fig. 8, *d*). These are semilunar or mitral cells with four to six ramifying horizontal processes projecting from their upper surface. These branches extend widely within the fifth sublayer.

(b) *The small type.* This is generally semilunar or cuboidal, and can be differentiated from the above cells by the fact that an extraordinarily large number of fine fibers arise from their upper surface. These fibers have only a few branches, but they are of enormous length. The appearance of these fibrils is reminiscent of a nerve fiber. They extend within the entire fifth sublayer and a good part of the fourth and third sublayers (Plate V, Fig. 9, *b*).

B. Bilayered and Multilayered Ganglion Cells

Just as in birds and reptiles, many types of these interesting cells can be found in mammals. The following are the types I encountered most frequently.

1. Cells which Arborize in the Second and Third Sublayers

Two types can be distinguished in this group: the giant type and the small type.

The giant type is very abundant, and it corresponds exactly to the bistratified or tristratified variety which I described in birds and reptiles (see Plate III, Fig. 6, *c* and Plate V, Fig. 1, *G*). The cell body is semilunar or mitral in shape. Two, three, or more stout processes arise from the upper surface of the cell, and these suddenly alter their course so as to form a plexus of thick fibers in the fourth sublayer. A large number of fibrils project from the thick branches of this horizontal plexus and ascend at a right angle to the second sublayer, forming a second dense plexus of varicose fibers (Plate V, Fig. 7, *f*).

In reptiles and birds, a third system of ramifications arises from these ganglion cells and lies within the third sublayer (Plate III, Fig. 6, *c*). In the mammals the middle plexus is absent.

The small type is very similar to the above giant type, except that the branches which form both horizontal plexuses are much more delicate and abundant (Plate V, Fig. 8, *i*).

2. Ganglion Cells which Ramify in Three Sublayers

I found only one cell of this type (Plate V, Fig. 7, *b*). It is small and pyriform, and has an ascending trunk which quickly breaks up into fine branches. These branches arrange themselves in three successive plexuses: one in the fifth, another in the third, and one in the second sublayer.

C. Diffuse Ganglion Cells

In the mammalian retina one consistently finds ganglion cell bodies whose protoplasmic branches are distributed throughout the entire inner plexiform layer without forming any horizontal plexus (Plate V, Fig. 9, *i*).

As the reader will see from my description of these ganglion cells, they have many complicated forms and connections. Nonetheless, they can be summarized in a very simple way: Every sublayer of the inner plexiform layer receives the terminal arborizations of one type of ganglion cell; the lower terminal clusters of the bipolar cells in turn make contact with them.

It must probably be assumed that even the narrowest and most individualized conduction paths through the retina are composed of a group of bipolar cells which transmit their impressions to *one* ganglion cell. The terminal arborization of the ganglion cells is very extensive in comparison to the lower terminal clusters of the bipolar cells, although there are also relative differences in the extent of the protoplasmic ramifications of different ganglion cells. Thus, it seems likely that the arborization of a ganglion cell makes contact with a rather large group of bipolar cells, receiving and transmitting their activity. The most diffuse conduction pathway probably transmits the activity of a large number of bipolar cells, perhaps via the diffuse or multilayered ganglion cells.

The multiplicity of plexuses or of contact surfaces in the inner plexiform layer is related to the number and thinness of the bipolar cells. It seems to me that the number of plexuses in the periphery of this layer is reduced to three where the bipolar layer becomes noticeably thinner.

Indeed, the large number of contact surfaces or horizontal plexuses in the inner plexiform layer appears to allow for a large number of rather distinct conduction pathways in a small area of the retina. One can easily understand that, if the inner plexiform layer had only *one* layer of contact specialized for containing all of the extensive ramifications of the two structures in the nervous conduction pathway (the clusters of the bipolars and the flat ramifications of the ganglion cells), the activation of individual points which are kept distinct in the visual cell layer would be confounded by general activation, and a large portion of the perceptual acuity would thus be lost.

The shape of the axis cylinder of the ganglion cells in the mammalian retina has been known for a long time. Corti[33] first demonstrated the continuity of this process with an optic nerve fiber. The old methods of sectioning, however, did not permit a clarification of the arrangement of the fine protoplasmic ramifications. Nonetheless, Ranvier[34] had already indicated the presence of horizontal plexuses at various levels within the inner plexiform layer of the frog. In discussing the effect of one-third alcohol and osmic acid on the cerebral plexus of the retina (the inner plexiform layer), Ranvier says:

> The granular substance within the layer swells, becomes more homogeneous and is less refractive, so that the nerve fibers contained in the layer are more easily identified in vertical sections through the retina. Also in this way the central process of the bipolar cells, the ramified process of the unipolar cells (spongioblasts), and the peripheral processes of the multipolar cells can be traced farther than in other preparations. It can also be observed that *all of these processes converge to form one plexus, or instead, a series of plexuses which are parallel to the surface of the retina and are interlinked with one another by fibrils which descend vertically and diagonally.*

We are indebted to Dogiel[35] for a detailed description of this arrangement in lower vertebrates, based on results obtained with the Ehrlich method. Furthermore, it seems that E. Baquis[36] succeeded in observing a similar arrangement, judging from the figure accompanying his text; however, it is not described in the text.

The stratification of the ganglion cells in mammals has been recently described, independently, by Dogiel[37] and by myself.[38] According to Dogiel, the ganglion cells in the human retina can be divided into the following three classes: (a) cells whose protoplasmic ramification spreads in the lower part of the inner plexiform layer (fifth sublayer), (b) cells which send their ramifications approximately to the middle part of the inner plexiform layer (probably my third sublayer), and (c) cells whose ramifications reach almost to the outer border of the inner plexiform layer (my second sublayer).

In examining Dogiel's figures it can be easily observed that he has stained only certain ganglion cells, since he mentions neither the single-layered cells of the first or fourth sublayers, nor any of the multilayered cells. At the level of arborization, Dogiel described anastomoses between filaments originating from cells of the same type. Such an arrangement had already been presumed by W. Krause[39] in the giant cells of the calf retina, which had been stained by the Cox method. For my part, *I have never been able to establish the existence of a net in any region of the retina,* although in horizontal sections I have seen protoplasmic ramifications of the ganglion cells that were stained quite beautifully and completely. The fibers interlace and also contact one another, but when viewed at high magnification the independence of these processes can always be established.

Do relationships exist between the giant ganglion cells and the giant spongioblasts? W. Krause has determined that in the cat and indeed, in almost all classes of vertebrates with the exception of the fish, for each giant ganglion cell there is a corresponding large spongioblast above it in the inner nuclear layer. To me this seems quite likely, but unfortunately it is not possible with either the Golgi or the Ehrlich method to provide any proof for it, since if the ganglion cells are stained in a section, the spongioblasts are not, and vice versa.

OPTIC NERVE FIBER LAYER

Fibers which Are Continuous with Ganglion Cells

We know that the fibers of the optic nerve layer are arranged in diverging bundles which become progressively thinner as they approach the ora serrata. The majority of nerve fibers are of slight or medium thickness. There are others, though, which are quite stout, and these are united three to four in a bundle; they are continuous with the giant ganglion cells.

All optic fibers have oval or roundish varicosities at variable distances, as Tartuferi has demonstrated.

The continuity of a rather considerable number of optic nerve fibers with the axis cylinders of the ganglion cells can be recognized easily in sections stained with methylene blue as well as in sections stained with chromium-silver and prepared according to the rolling-up procedure.

Centrifugal Fibers

These are most difficult to stain in the mammal. I have stained them a few times in the dog retina. They are very fine and ascend vertically through the inner plexiform layer to the amacrine cell layer, where they end freely in a varicose ramification of fine ascending branches which make contact with the cell body and the descending trunk of the spongioblasts (Plate V, Fig. 2, *j*).

In addition to the centrifugal fibers, I have also seen other nerve fibers which are of equal fineness. They originate in the optic fiber layer and ascend obliquely through the inner plexiform layer, so as then to take a horizontal course at various levels within this layer. I have not succeeded in discovering their termination, so I remain unclear as to their destination (Plate V, Fig. 2, *m*). These fibers do not stain with methylene blue. It is only by using the double impregnation procedure that I have succeeded in seeing them.

NEUROGLIA

Two types of structural elements can be distinguished in the retina: Müller fibers or epithelial cells, and spider cells ("Spinnenzellen," "cellules en araignée") or true neuroglial cells.

The Müller Fibers

These are well-known to many investigators, since they can be recognized just as well with one-third alcohol as with Schiefferdecker's mixture. With chromium-silver they stain very often, perhaps too often, and it is not unusual that their staining hinders the observation of other elements. Moreover, with this stain a definite difference can be established between the reaction of nerve cells and Müller fibers. If Müller fibers are well stained, most of the nerve cells and nerve fibers are not stained at all, or the impregnation is quite incomplete.

The arrangement of the epithelial cells differs little from that in the frog or teleost fish. I would add only the following:

1. At the level of the nuclei of the visual cells, the extensions of the Müller fibers completely surround the individual cells, thereby rendering lateral conduction of an impulse impossible.
2. At the level of the outer plexiform layer lateral extensions are absent or insignificant; thus, the contiguity between fibers within this layer is not impeded.
3. At the level of the inner nuclear layer the protoplasmic

extensions of the epithelial cells are rather short, thereby incompletely isolating the bipolars and amacrine cells.
4. The collateral branches given off in the inner plexiform layer are very fine, granular, and wavy. They end freely, leaving horizontal spaces between them. The spaces contain the plexuses formed by the parallel ramifications of ganglion cells and amacrine cells.
5. The extensions destined for the ganglion cell layer are very short and thick; sometimes they appear only as irregular thickenings.

Just as in the other classes of vertebrates, the foot of the epithelial cell is frequently bifurcated, allowing a nerve bundle to pass between. On approaching the optic disk, where the optic nerve fiber layer is most developed, the end-feet are very often divided into two or even three branches. In addition to the usual extensions, it is not uncommon to find a few projections arising from the protoplasm which surrounds the nucleus; these sink into the inner plexiform layer where they end freely (Plate VI, Fig. 5, *a*).

Spider Cells

If a retinal section stained with carmine or hemotoxylin is examined, certain oval or roundish nuclei surrounded by granular protoplasm can be observed in the optic fiber layer. The similarity of these cells with the cells which lie among the optic nerve fascicles supports the notion of Schwalbe,[40] Golgi and Manfredi,[41] and Borysiekiewicz[42] *et al.* that these are true neuroglial cells.

Staining with chromium-silver completely confirms this assumption and makes it possible to add a few details which had not been revealed by the older methods.

According to their location, the neuroglial cells can be placed in two categories: the cells of the ganglion cell layer, and the cells of the optic fiber layer.

The former have a triangular, roundish, or semilunar cell body (Plate VI, Fig. 12, *i*). A fiber, or a bundle of very fine vertical fibrils, very often proceeds from their upper surface and then disappears in the lower third of the inner plexiform layer.

Two or three bundles of delicate fibrils project from their lower surface, the majority of which take the same direction as the optic fibers and terminate among them.

The neuroglia cells of the optic fiber layer (Plate VI, Fig. 12, f, h, j, g) occur in a number of shapes. In general those which lie in the neighborhood of the internal limiting membrane are triangular and characterized by the fact that most of their processes arise from an external protoplasmic branch. Those cells which are situated among the bundles of the nerve fibers are stellate and send processes out in all directions. Most of these processes, however, travel in the direction of the nerve bundles (Plate VI, Fig. 12, j).

The fibers of the neuroglia cells are very long, thin, and granular. With the Golgi method they appear light coffee-brown. Near their origin they are usually arranged together in thick bundles. Sometimes a few processes extend from the external surface of the cell to reach the inner plexiform layer and branch repeatedly (Plate VI, Fig. 12, h).

It is not unusual that the protoplasm of the cells is arranged in lamellae with concave contours between the bundles of fibrils. This arrangement was first noted by Golgi and Manfredi, using the older methods.

The optic nerve impregnated with chromium-silver shows true neuroglial cells, as Leber,[43] Schwalbe,[44] and Petrone[45] have demonstrated with different methods. The cells are especially remarkable in their considerable volume and the enormous length of their processes. Such cells can be subdivided into (a) cells which lie in the middle of the optic nerve, and (b) cells which lie in the area of the optic disk.

The first type is stellate and has very stout processes which ramify repeatedly. Their fibrils are long and collect in a bundle which courses laterally; they divide the optic fiber bundle completely by forming an extraordinarily abundant and complicated lattice around it.

The second type is small and irregularly-shaped, having fine processes packed very close together. Most of these processes are directed forward. The cells which touch the surface of the optic disk are entirely comparable with the anterior cells of the optic fiber layer.

As noted in previous chapters, spider cells are found in the optic nerve of all vertebrates. It is noteworthy that the processes of these cells become more dense and lamellated as one ascends the phylogenetic scale of vertebrates.

REFERENCES

1. Schiefferdecker, P.: Studien zur vergleichenden Histologie der Retina. *Arch. f. mikrosk. Anat.*, 1886 (28), 305-396.
2. Borysiekiewicz, M.: Untersuchungen über den feineren Bau der Netzhaut. Leipzig u. Wien, 1887.
3. Kuhnt, H.: Histologische Studien an der menschlichen Netzhaut. *Jenaische Zeitschr. f. Naturwissensch.*, 1890 (24), p. 177.
4. Lenox, R.: Beobachtungen über die Histologie der Netzhaut mittelst der Weigert'schen Färbungsmethode. *von Graefe's Arch. f. Ophthal.*, 1886 (32), 1-8.
5. Tartuferi, F.: Sull'anatomia della retina. *Intern. Monatsschr. f. Anat. u. Physiol.*, 1887 (4), 421-441.
6. Dogiel, A.: Über die nervösen Elemente in der Retina des Menschen. Erste Mitteilung. *Archiv f. mikrosk, Anat.*, 1891 (38), 317-344.
7. Schwalbe, G.: *Lehrbuch der Anatomie der Sinnesorgane.* Erlangen, 1887.
8. Ranvier, L.: *Traité technique d'histologie.* Paris, 1875-1882.
9. Ramón y Cajal, S.: Notas preventivas sobre la retina y gran simpático de los mamíferos. *Gac. Sanit. d. Barcelona,* 10 December, 1891.
10. Baquis, E.: La retina della faina. *Anat. Anz.* 1890 (5), 366-371.
11. Krause, W.: Die Retina. *Intern. Monatsschr. f. Anat. u. Physiol.* 1891 (8), 414-415.
12. Schultze, M.: Zur Anatomie und Physiologie der Retina. *Arch. f. mikrosk. Anat.*, 1866 (2) 175-286.

    Schultze, M.: Sehorgan. I. Die Retina. In Stricker, S. (Ed.): *Handbuch der Lehre von den Geweben des Menschen und der Tiere.* Leipzig, 1872, Vol. II, p. 992.

    Hannover, A.: La rétine de l'homme et des vertébrés. Paris, 1876, 164 pp.
13. Ramón y Cajal, S.: Sur la morphologie et les connexions des éléments de la rétine des oiseaux. *Anat. Anz.*, 1889 (4), 111-121.
14. Dogiel, A.: Über die nervösen Elemente in der Retina des Menschen. Erste Mitteilung. *Arch. f. mikrosk. Anat.*, 1891 (38), 320.
15. Dogiel, A.: Über die nervösen Elemente in der Retina des Menschen. Zweite Mitteilung. *Arch. f. mikrosk. Anat.* 1892 (40), 29-38.

    Merkel, F., and Zuckerkandl, E.: Sinnesorgane. *Ergeb. d. Anat. u. Entwickelungsgesch.*, 1892 (2), 253.

Waldeyer, W.: Ergebnisse der Anatomie und Entwickelungsgeschichte. (Kritiken u. Referaten) *Berliner klin. Wochenschr.,* 1894 (31), 249-250.

16. Merkel, F.: Über die menschliche Retina. *von Graefe's Arch. f. Ophthal.,* 1876 (22), 1-25.
17. Kölliker, A.: *Handbuch der Gewebelehre des Menschen,* 5th ed. Leipzig, 1867.
18. Manfredi, and Golgi, C.: Annotazioni istologishe sulla retina del cavallo. *Giorn. d. Accad. d. med. d. Torino,* 1872 (12), 289-351.
19. Rivolta, S.: Dello strato di cellule multipolari che formano lo strato intergranuloso o intermedio nella retina del cavallo. *Giorn. d. Anat. Fisiol. e Patol. d. Anim.,* 1871 (3), 185-200.
20. Schwalbe, G.: Mikroskopische Anatomie des Sehnerven, der Netzhaut, und des Glaskörpers. In von Graefe, A. and Saemisch, T. (Eds.): *Handbuch der ges. Augenheilk.* Leipzig, 1874, Vol. I, pp. 321-479.
21. Dogiel, A.: Über die Retina des Menschen. *Intern. Monatsschr. f. Anat. u. Physiol.,* 1884 (1), 143-151.
22. Ravier, D.: *Traité technique d'histologie.* Paris, 1882.
23. Krause, W.: *Allgemeine und mikroskopische Anatomie.* Hannover, 1876.
24. Schiefferdecker, P.: Studien zur vergleichenden Histologie der Retina. *Arch. f. mikrosk. Anat.,* 1886 (28), 362 ff.
25. Ramón y Cajal, S.: Pequeñas contribuciones al conocimiento del sistema nervioso. III. La retina de las batracios y reptiles. 20 August, 1891.
26. Ramón y Cajal, S.: Notas preventivas sobre la retina y gran simpático de los mamíferos. *Gaz. Sanit. de Barcelona,* 10 December, 1891.
27. Dogiel, A.: Über die nervösen Elemente in der Retina des Menschen. *Arch. f. mikrosk. Anat.,* 1891 (38), 317-344.
28. Retzius, G.: Zur Kenntniss des Nervensystems der Crustacean. *Biol. Unters., Neue Folge,* 1890 (1), 1-50.
29. von Lenhossék, M.: Ursprung, Verlauf, und Endigung der sensibeln Nervenfasern bei Lumbricus. *Arch. f. mikrosk. Anat.,* 1892 (39), 102-136.
30. Nagel, A.: Die fettige Degeneration der Netzhaut. *von Graefe's Archiv f. Ophthal.,* 1860 (6), 218.
31. Müller, H.: Anatomisch-physiologische Untersuchungen über die Retina des Menschen und der Wirbeltiere. *Zeitschr. f. wissensch. Zool.,* 1857 (8), 1-122.
32. Borysiekiewicz, M.: Untersuchungen über den feineren Bau der Netzhaut. Leipzig u. Wien, 1887.
33. Corti, A.: Beitrag zur Anatomie der Retina. *Arch. f. Anat., Physiol., u. wissensch. Med.,* 1850, p. 273.

    Corti, A.: Histologische Untersuchungen angestellt an einem Elephanten. *Zeitschr. f. wissensch. Zool.,* 1954 (5), 84.
34. Ranvier, L.: *Traité technique d'histologie.* Paris, 1882, p. 978.
35. Dogiel, A.: Über das Verhalten der nervösen Elemente in der Retina

der Ganoiden, Reptilien, Vögel, und Säugetiere. *Anat. Anz.,* 1888 (3), 133-143.
36. Baquis, E.: La retina della faina. *Anat. Anz.,* 1890 (5), 366-371.
37. Dogiel, A.: Über die nervösen Elemente in der Retina des Menschen. Erste Mitteilung. *Arch. f. mikrosk. Anat.,* 1891 (38), 317-344.
38. Ramón y Cajal, S.: Notas preventivas sobre la retina y gran simpático de los mamíferos. *Gac. Sanit. de Barcelona.* 10 December, 1891.
39. Krause, W.: Die Retina. *Intern. Monatsschr. f. Anat. u. Physiol.,* 1891 (8), 414-415.
40. Schwalbe, G.: Mikroskopische Anatomie des Sehnerven, der Netzhaut, und des Glaskörpers. In von Graefe, A., and Saemisch, T. (Eds.): *Handbuch d. ges. Augenheilk.* Leipzig, 1874, Vol. I, pp. 321-479.
41. Manfredi, and Golgi, C.: Annotazioni istologiche sulla retina del cavallo. *Giorn. d. Accad. d. med. d. Torino,* 1872 (12), 289-351.
42. Borysiekiewicz, M.: Untersuchungen über den feineren Bau der Netzhaut. Leipzig u. Wien, 1887.
43. Leber, T.: Beiträge zur Kenntnis der atrophischen Veränderungen des Sehnerven nebst Bemerkungen über die normale Struktur der Nerven. *von Graefe's Arch. f. Ophthal.,* 1868 (14), Abt. 2, p. 169.
44. Schwalbe, G.: Mikroskopische Anatomie des Sehnerven, der Netzhaut, und des Glaskörpers. In von Graefe, A., and Saemisch, T. (Eds.): *Handbuch d. ges. Augenheilk.* Leipzig, 1874, Vol. I, pp. 321-479.
45. Petrone, L.: Sur la structure des nerfs cerébro-rachidiens. *Intern. Monatsschr. f. Anat. u. Physiol.,* 1888 (5), 39-47.

Chapter VIII

THE FOVEA CENTRALIS

EVEN though my investigations on the structure of the fovea centralis have not been completed, I would like to report briefly my findings in passerine birds (house sparrow, green finch, chaffinch, etc.) and in the reptile (chameleon). In my opinion these animals are especially suited for resolving the fascinating problems which still exist in this area.

THE FOVEA CENTRALIS IN SPARROWS*

The Visual Cell Layer

Only cones are found in and around the fovea centralis; these cones are longer and finer than those in other regions of the retina (Plate VI, Fig. 16, *a*). At the junction of the outer and inner segments, a roundish swelling which corresponds to a colored oil droplet can be seen often.

The Layer of Visual Cell Nuclei

This layer is very thick and is composed of many rows of cone nuclei. The majority of the nuclei are located in the lower half of the layer; the upper half is composed mainly of ascending fibers of the cones. These fibers are straight in the central part of the fovea (Plate VI, Fig. 16, *c*); however, in the more lateral region they course very obliquely and often are concave outward near the outer limiting membrane (Plate VI, Fig. 16, *d*). The descending fiber of the cones terminate in the outer plexiform layer with a large conical or ellipsoidal swelling, having either no basilar filaments at all (Plate VI, Fig. 16, *f*) or only a few very short and seemingly rudimentary fibrils. These terminal swellings are arranged in two layers.

---

* The fovea centralis of the bird was discovered by H. Müller[1] and thoroughly described in his publications: "Uber das Vorkommen einer dem gelben Fleck der Retina entsprechenden Stelle bei Tieren." *Würzb. naturw. Zeitschr.*, 1861, Bd. II. Also Über das Vorhandensein zweier Foveae in der Netzhaut vieler Vogelaugen." *Zehender's klin. Monatsbl.*, 1863. (Greeff's note)

Bipolar Cell Layer

The bipolar cell layer in this area attains a much greater thickness than in any other portion of the retina because of the extraordinary number of bipolar cells and spongioblasts which it contains.

The bipolar cells are oriented vertically in the central part of the fovea. However, the more peripheral their location, the more obliquely they lie (Plate VI, Fig. 16, h). It is this fact, which is so well known to investigators who have studied the fovea in different classes of vertebrates (Müller, Schultze, Kuhnt, Krause, Chiewitz, etc.), which is one of the most important characteristics of this retinal region. This oblique orientation remains over an area of several square millimeters.

The cell bodies of the bipolars lie in the lower part of the inner nuclear layer, just above the spongioblasts. Their ascending process extends to the outer plexiform layer where it forms a tiny, flat, and completely rudimentary arborization (Plate VI, Fig. 18, g). The small size of this arborization permits connection with only a single terminal swelling of a cone. In the central part of the fovea the arborization is often replaced by a nodule which touches the lower surface of the cone pedicle. Sometimes this nodule sends out a short ascending fiber which runs alongside the pedicle of the cone. Landolt clubs are never found, or at least I have not been able to stain them. Upon arrival at the inner plexiform layer, the descending process of the bipolar cell travels through this layer vertically and terminates in a restricted varicose arborization lying below the fourth sublayer. I cannot say whether the bipolar cells lying in the thinnest part of the retina behave in the same manner, because I have not yet stained their descending processes.*

---

*In my most recent investigations I believe I have shown that the descending processes of the bipolar cells do not send out any collateral branches. At least I can affirm that if such collaterals do exist, they are never made visible by staining with chromium-silver. If this fact were established, then the doctrine of individual nervous conduction (i.e. the conduction of an impulse from one neuron to another neuron lying deeper) would have new support for the region of the fovea centralis. (1894 edition)

The amacrine cells at the edges of the fovea, which were the only ones evident in my sections, are very abundant. They are characterized by the relatively small extent of their arborizations, which are given off in the inner plexiform layer. In the region of the fovea these arborizations form a considerable number of plexuses, at least seven.

Ganglion Cell Layer

I have not been able to stain the ganglion cells of the central part of the fovea; however, at the edges of the fovea they stain very beautifully. The most important characteristic of these cells is the smallness of their ascending clusters, which lie in the various sublayers of the inner plexiform layer. The ganglion cells which I have been able to observe up to this time are, without exception, the single-layered type of cell (Plate VI, Fig. 16, j, l).*

THE FOVEA CENTRALIS IN THE CHAMELEON

The fovea centralis of this reptile has already been studied by H. Müller.[2] It is very easy to see, and thus it is very suitable for studying the arrangement of the cells in this region. The

---

*In staining recently undertaken on the green finch retina I have found almost all cell types seen at other locations in the retina to occur at the edges of the fovea. These include (a) nerve or ganglion cells with rather extensive protoplasmic terminal arborizations which lie within the second or third sublayer of the inner plexiform layer, (b) nervous spongioblasts, or Dogiel cells, (c) amacrine cells which extend to the second, third, or fifth sublayer. The extent of the terminal arborizations of these cells appear to decrease slightly only in that region nearest the center of the fovea. At the edges of the fovea they have normal dimensions. This finding brought me to think that perhaps the lower terminal cluster of the bipolar cells articulates only with the center of a flat arborization of a ganglion cell, whereas the rest of this arborization receives the clusters of the amacrine cells exclusively. This might be the best way to account for the individualized conduction through the retina of a stimulus received by a single cone. Such an idea, however, requires further investigation. Perhaps a comparative count of the number of bipolar cell nuclei on the one hand, and of the ganglion cell nuclei on the other, over a rather large area in and around the fovea would provide support for this hypothesis, i.e. if the count yielded a roughly equal quantity of both types of cells here. (1894 edition)

chameleon's fovea centralis is surrounded by a large swelling of the retina, where very good staining of the visual cells occurs.*

Visual Cell Layer

The cones, the only elements which occur here, are extremely delicate and long. In the central part of the retina, the inner segments have the same thickness as the outer segments. The pigment cells are well developed and surround the cones completely. The lamellar extensions which arise from the outer limiting membrane are also very long.

Layer of Visual Cell Nuclei

This layer is very thick, especially in the area of the foveal pit (Plate VI, Fig. 15). It can be divided into two subzones: (a) the outer subzone, which contains almost exclusively the cell bodies and nuclei of the cones, and (b) the inner subzone, which is broader and contains the descending fibers of these cells.

At the level of the outer subzone, the fibers of the cones run almost vertically or slightly obliquely, but as soon as they reach the inner subzone they become quite varicose and follow a course which is so oblique, that together they give the impression of a layer of horizontal nerve fibers. They retain this orientation throughout the retina, and it is even exaggerated in the most peripheral regions. The terminal swellings of the cone fibers are small and have no basilar processes (Plate VI, Fig. 15). They are arranged in two strata in the outer plexiform layer, where they make contact with two corresponding rows of bipolar cell clusters.

Bipolar Cells

These are very small and very numerous, especially at the edges of the foveal pit. At the deepest part of the fovea their

---

*While this (1894) volume was being printed, I obtained a monograph from W. Krause[3]: "Die Retina der Reptilien" (Fortsetzung). *Intern. Monatsschr. f. Anat. u. Physiol.*, Heft 2, 1892, Bd. X. Although Krause has used techniques different than mine, the results which he obtained agree in many respects with my own results. This is an excellent study of the chameleon retina. (Cajal's 1894 footnote)

course is vertical and somewhat wavy (Plate VI, Fig. 15, *c*), while at the edge of the fovea and in the area surrounding it, they travel more and more obliquely and radially. These cells, however, are not as obliquely oriented as the fibers from the cone nuclei.

The ascending process of the bipolar cell terminates in the outer plexiform layer with an exceptionally small arborization that is applied very closely to the base of a cone terminal swelling (Plate VI, Fig. 15, *e*). At some distance from the fovea, these arborizations increase progressively in extent and surround the terminal swellings of two or three cone fibers. As I mentioned previously, the clusters of the bipolar cells are arranged in two layers, so as to make contact with the two rows of cone terminal swellings. In regions somewhat removed from the fovea, the terminal swellings of the cones have very short radial collateral branches.

The descending process of the bipolar cells terminates in an ordinary manner within the inner plexiform layer, i.e. with a collateral terminal arborization of very narrow extent.

The Amacrine and Ganglion Cells

These are abundant at the edges of the fovea and are also characterized by the smallness of their terminal arborization. However, the reduction in the extent of the protoplasmic arborizations of both types of cells is never as obvious as that seen in the terminal swellings of the cones and the ascending clusters of the bipolars. As we will see later, this fact is important because it explains a phenomenon which at first glance appears peculiar: namely, the oblique course of the visual cells and the bipolar cells.

In the epithelial cells I have discovered two facts of some interest. First, the division into descending branches (terminal clusters) does not occur at the level of the vitreal border of the inner plexiform layer but rather within the inner plexiform layer itself (Plate VI, Fig. 15). Second, the cell bodies of the epithelial cells bifurcate in the outer half of the layer of visual cell nuclei. One of the branches courses diagonally or horizontally and travels over an enormously wide extent along with the descending fibers of the cones. Finally it runs vertically and terminates with a descending cluster (Plate VI, Fig. 15, g). In the central part of the fovea, as well as at the edges, the Müller fibers are shorter and not as slanted because of the fact that they always follow the direction of the descending processes of the nuclei in the outer nuclear layer.

In summary, the fovea centralis of birds and reptiles is characterized by the thinness of the cones, the smallness of the ascending arborizations of the bipolar cells, and the absence of basilar appendages on the terminal swellings of the cells in the outer nuclear layer. A stimulus received by a cone maintains its individuality on its course through the inner nuclear layer, since the terminal swelling of the cones makes contact with only one tiny terminal cluster of the bipolar cells.

The decrease in diameter of the cones, which allows more visual cells to be accommodated within a given area of the retina, accounts for all of the modifications which occur in other layers, especially in the vicinity of the fovea. These modifications include the considerable thickness of the outer nuclear layer, the increase in the number of bipolars, the relative smallness of the bipolars, and the very large size of the amacrine and ganglion cell layer.

The oblique course of the visual cells and the bipolar cells is determined by two conditions: first, a virtually complete or total absence of spongioblasts and ganglion cells in the deep part of the fovea; second, and this is the more important reason, a certain area of contact between bipolars and ganglion cells is necessary (like the concentric plexuses of the inner plexiform layer). In order to have the necessary contact surface between cells in the fovea, not only the edges of the fovea but also the adjacent parts must be pushed away. The thinner and more numerous the cones, the larger must be the retinal zone in which the cone fibers from the fovea centralis and the bipolar cells extend and make contact. As I noted above, the reduction in the contact surface at the level of the inner plexiform layer is much less than that at the level of the outer plexiform layer (i.e. between the clusters of the bipolar cells and the terminal swellings of the cones).

Although I have not yet concluded my investigations in this area, I believe I can say that the fovea of man and other vertebrates is constructed in the manner just described above. In the human retina the slant of the cone fibers is quite pronounced, and two subzones can be easily recognized in the outer nuclear layer, just as in the chameleon.

REFERENCES

1. Müller, H.: Über das Vorkommen einer dem gelben Fleck der Retina entsprechenden Stelle bei Tieren. *Würzb. naturw. Zeitschr.*, 1861 (2), 139.

    Müller, H.: Über das Vorhandensein zweier Foveae in der Netzhaut vieler Vogelaugen. *Klin. Monatsbl. f. Augenheilk.*, 1863 (1), 438.
2. Müller, H.: Über das Auge des Chamäleons, mit vergleichenden Bemerkungen. *Würzb. naturw. Zeitschr.*, 1862 (3), 10.
3. Krause, W.: Die Retina der Reptilien (Fortsetzung). *Intern. Monatsschr. f. Anat. u. Physiol.*, 1892 (10), 12, 33, 68.

Chapter IX

THE DEVELOPMENT OF RETINAL CELLS

THE development of the retina has been the object of study for a number of investigators, notably Babuchin,[1] Löwe,[2] Ogneff,[3] Bellonci,[4] Koganeï,[5] and H. Chievitz.[6]

My own research on this problem is not yet finished, so I will restrict myself here to a brief description of the results obtained with the Golgi method concerning the metamorphosis of Müller fibers and some nerve cells.

My observations were made with embryos of the mouse, rabbit, calf, and chicken. I was able to study the retina only after the inner plexiform layer and the ganglion cell layer were differentiated. My attempts at staining during earlier stages, e.g. when the inner nuclear layers are continuous with the ganglion cell layer so that no demarcation line can be seen, have so far been unsuccessful.

THE EPITHELIAL CELLS

In sections of a very young retina, the structural cells stain exclusively (Plate VII, Fig. 1, d). Their shape is completely reminiscent of the form of the epithelial cells in the fetal medulla. They are elongated and fusiform, with oval cell bodies surrounding the nucleus. They have two delicate processes, an ascending and a descending one, which terminate on the retinal surface with conical swellings. The fact that the embryonic retina has fusiform cells whose processes reach the two membrane surfaces has already been described by Babuchin.

In the first stage of development, the cell bodies of the Müller fibers and hence, their nuclei, are scattered throughout the entire thickness of the retina with the exception of the ganglion cell layer and the optic fiber layer (Plate VII, Fig. 1). However, as this membrane increases in thickness and as the anatomical differentiation of the layers proceeds, the nuclei migrate toward the central part of the retina near the inner plexiform layer, i.e. to the region which will later become the inner nuclear layer, where they definitely settle (Plate VII, Fig. 3).

As the development of the Müller fibers progresses, their contours become more irregular. Their upper endings, which are initially simple, later may bifurcate so as to form the peripheral clusters like those of the radial or epithelial cells seen in the fetal brain, but in a less complex configuration (Plate VII, Fig. 2, f).

Ultimately the epithelial cells increase in thickness. Lamellar expansions arise from their central and peripheral processes. Their outer extremity, which is transformed into a flat lamella, gives off fine fibers which penetrate among the developing visual cells. In the bird embryo, where I have studied this phase extensively, it can be seen that the lateral lamellae of the Müller fibers begin at the level of the spongioblasts. At the level of the outer nuclei the formation of lamellae is preceded by the construction of a roundish or oval protoplasmic mass, a type of reserve material from which the collateral branches later develop (Plate VII, Fig. 3, a).

In the chick and lizard embryo I have been able to establish an interesting fact regarding the appearance of the terminal division of the deep processes of the Müller fibers. As is well known, in these animals the Müller fibers divide into a bundle of descending fibrils at the level of the amacrine cell layer. These fibrils terminate at the inner limiting membrane with a conical thickening. In the embryo this division into fibrils starts at the ganglion cell layer and continues later to the spongioblast layer via a type of longitudinal fissure.

THE LAYER OF GANGLION CELLS AND OPTIC FIBERS

These layers are the first to be differentiated in very young embryos, as has been noted by other workers, namely Kölliker[7] and Chievitz.[6] Only when these layers are formed does the inner plexiform layer appear.

In a mouse embryo some 15 cm in length I did succeed in staining ganglion cells, even though this layer was not yet fully developed (Plate VII, Fig. 1). The first thing one notices is that these cells still lie at a considerable distance from the optic fiber layer and are not yet arranged in a regular layer. Their shape, especially that of the youngest cells, is entirely similar to the neuroblasts of His.[8] They are pyriform with a descending foot that is continuous with a fiber of the optic nerve (Plate VII, Fig. 1, *a*). The more developed ganglion cells exhibit a few rudimentary protoplasmic processes, which may be divided into ascending and descending processes. The former arise from the upper surface of the cell body, bifurcate and terminate in the upper layer with very thick varicosities. The latter—one, two, or three in number—proceed either from the lower part of the cell body or from the base of the nerve process and pass into the optic fiber layer where they end freely (Plate VII, Fig. 1, *g*).

Later the upper processes divide several times, as can be seen in Plate VII, Fig. 2, *e*, and they form a complicated horizontal arborization. The lower processes, on the other hand, meander for a while among the optic fibers, but ultimately they atrophy and disappear completely.

It can be seen that the development of the protoplasmic branches in the retina proceeds in almost the same manner as in the spinal cord of the chick embryo where von Lenhossék[9] and I myself[10] were able to follow all the phases of development in the neuroblasts of His.

The optic nerve fibers stain very easily in the embryonic retina, and they can be easily traced in the optic nerve. Unfortunately I have not been able to stain them in earlier stages of development when they are still growing. Thus, I cannot take a position in the debate conducted for so long between W. Müller,[11] who is of the opinion that upon leaving the retina, the optic fibers grow out from the stalk of the optic vesicle, and W. His,[12] Kölliker,[13] and others, who suppose growth to occur in the opposite manner, i.e. from the brain to the optic vesicle. If one may reason by analogy on such a difficult subject, then I would like to say that both views can be sustained. On the basis of the latest theory of His on the growth of the axis cylinders of the neuroblasts, and also the most recent discoveries of the termination of nerve fibers, it seems reasonable to suggest that those retinal fibers which arise from ganglion cells grow in a centripetal direction, while those fibers whose origin lies in the optic center grow in a centrifugal direction.*

Plate VII, Figure 4 shows an anteroposterior section through the eye of a mouse embryo. In C a very considerable retinal fold, which has been described by Kölliker, can be seen. The Müller fibers appear quite twisted and thick. The prisms of the crystalline lens often stain with chromium-silver and exhibit rough contours, although they never have connecting processes. Several central prisms have already lost their nucleus.

Although my observations on the other layers of the retina are still incomplete, I would like to mention some of them.

THE AMACRINE CELLS

These cells appear at the same time as the ganglion cells. The development of their lower clusters marks the beginning of the formation of the inner plexiform layer. The fibers of the terminal arborizations of the lower cluster are very short, thick, and very varicose. They are associated with the branches of the ascending clusters of the ganglion cells. In a chick on the fourteenth day of incubation, the nervous spongioblasts are completely differentiated (Plate VII, Fig. 3, u), and the various types of amacrine cells can already be recognized.

THE BIPOLAR CELLS

In a chick embryo of thirteen days incubation the bipolar cells are clearly visible (Plate VII, Fig. 3, m), but their upper and lower clusters are still very short and have a granular appearance. The Landolt clubs are relatively thick.†

---

*This opinion was formulated by Müller and has been confirmed in recent years by me (1906) and also by Held and Tello, all of whom employed the neurofibrillar method. (1933 edition)

† Very recently I succeeded in staining retinae from the ninth and tenth days of incubation. They are already quite well developed, as the inner plexiform layer is already formed, though very thin. In such retinae the bipolar cells look just like those found in the olfactory mucous membrane. They have an elongated cell body, which is almost completely occupied by the nucleus, and two processes: (a) an ascending one which is thick and virtually straight, and ends in a

(Continued on page 144)

In the retina of even younger embryos, e.g. that represented in Plate VII, Figure 1 from a 15 mm mouse embryo, it is impossible to distinguish the bipolar cells from the visual cells and even from incompletely stained Müller fibers. I suspect, however, that certain fusiform cells located at different levels in the outer half of the retina are bipolar cells. These cells are characterized by their short descending process which terminates in a swelling (Plate VII, Fig. 2, *b*). The outer process reaches the outer limiting membrane. I must hasten to add, however, that since the outer nuclear layer and the outer plexiform layer are not yet differentiated at this time, I cannot be completely confident that these fusiform elements are really bipolar cells, especially since they seem to have the same properties as certain other elements which lie very near the outer limiting membrane and which might well be the rudimentary visual cells or the proliferated cells ("cellules proliférantes") of Koganeï and Chievitz (Plate VII, Fig. 2, *g*).

VISUAL CELLS

My studies of the rods and cones and their nuclei are even less precise. In the embryo of the newborn rabbit the outer nuclear layer is already formed (Plate VII, Fig. 12); it may be seen to be separated from the inner nuclear layer by the outer plexiform layer. The outer nuclear layer contains two types of cells: those which have a single ascending process and those which

---

(Continued from page 143)

varicosity at the level of the outer limiting membrane, and (b) a very delicate descending process which closely resembles a nerve fiber and terminates in the inner (but still rudimentary) plexiform zone with a small swelling. This swelling is more or less regular in shape, but shows no tendency to branch, as is later the case. In several bipolar cells situated at the level of the newly formed outer plexiform layer, one or two small thickenings can be seen on the thick or outer process. These thickenings represent the rudimentary Anlage of the flat ramifications which will be formed within the strata of the outer plexiform layer. On the eleventh day of incubation, a few ramifications of this type are already clearly delineated. Thus, we see that the formation of the Landolt clubs precedes that of the arborizations of the outer plexiform layer (which arise from secondary branches), and that in their primitive Anlage the bipolar cells of the retina are quite comparable to the bipolar cells of the spinal ganglion and of the olfactory mucous membrane. (1894 edition)

have two processes—an ascending and a descending one. The latter type of descending process terminates freely with a very irregular swelling in the outer plexiform layer. It is my opinion that all these nuclei belong to the rods, and that the cone nuclei did not stain with chromium-silver.

In the retina of a chick on the thirteenth day of incubation, the outer nuclei are already formed, and both types of cone fibers can be observed: straight fibers and diagonal fibers (Plate VII, Fig. 3, e). The rods and cones themselves are represented as very short hyalin outgrowths, as Kölliker, Babuchin, Chievitz, and others have noted. They grow from the peripheral ends of the fibers which arise from the nuclei. They do not stain with chromium-silver.*

THE HORIZONTAL CELLS

These cells stain very beautifully in the retina of the newborn rabbit (Plate VII, Fig. 12). They are semilunar and have two thick horizontal processes which ramify in the middle of the outer plexiform layer. Two cell types can be distinguished: cells with a descending protoplasmic process, and cells with only horizontal processes. The later are more numerous, and in horizontal sections made through the retina they can be seen to form a tightly-meshed net by intimate contact of their protoplasmic processes.

In the study of the development of the retina and the nervous centers, I have often asked myself the following question:

---

*In the retina of a chick embryo fourteen to fifteen days after incubation all the nerve cells are almost completely formed. In my most recent sections I could see almost all types of spongioblasts and ganglion cells. The amacrine cells are especially beautiful with their stellate clusters situated in the second sublayer. The radial fibrils travel along a virtually straight course, with nearly all of them terminating at the same distance with a roundish and rather considerable nodosity. Moreover, the ganglion cells of the second sublayer (Plate V, Fig. 1, E, G) are already very clearly developed. On the same sections I saw a nerve fiber which arose from the optic fiber layer, traversed the inner plexiform and inner nuclear layers, and having arrived at the outer plexiform zone, took a horizontal direction and could be followed even further. In its passage through the inner plexiform layer it gave off a collateral branch which coursed horizontally. I cannot say what significance these fibers have. They can be seen in mature batrachians and mammals, but only rarely. (1894 edition)

How does the mechanical development of the nerve fibers occur, and wherein lies that marvelous power which enables the nerve fibers from very distant cells to make contact directly with certain other nerve cells of the mesoderm or ectoderm without going astray or taking a roundabout course?

His has concerned himself with this important question[14] and is of the following opinion: The axis cylinder of the neuroblasts, whether in the medulla or in the mesoderm, always follows the path of least resistance. That resistance is offered by bone, cartilage, connective tissue, etc. which are found along the route of growing nerves. This accounts for the major part of the phenomenon.

Without wanting to deny the importance of such a mechanical influence, especially in the growth of the nerve fibers from the retina to the brain and vice versa, I believe that one could also think of processes like the phenomenon called Pfeffer's chemotaxis,[15] whose influences on the leukocytes was established by Massart and Bordet,[16] Gabritschewsky,[17] Buchner,[18] and Metchnikoff.[19] Metchnikoff has explained the union of the growth points of the embryonic vessels by chemotaxis.*

If a chemotaxic sensitivity in the neuroblasts is assumed, then it must be supposed that these cells are capable of amoeboid movement and are responsive to certain substances secreted by cells of the epithelium or mesoderm. The processes of the neuroblasts become oriented by chemical stimulation, and move toward the secretion products of certain cells.

The first of these two characteristics has already been demonstrated in the beautiful studies of His and my own work on the mode of growth of the cells of the spinal ganglion. These cells, which are initially bipolar in all vertebrates, ultimately become monopolar in the frog, reptile, bird, and mammal by virtue of a stalk which forms at the expense of the cell body and

---

*See the modern theories of the development of nerve fibers (normal and pathological) in the reports of Harrison, Forssman, Held, Ariëns-Kappers, Marinesco, Tello, and Cajal. Metchnikoff's exposition is detailed in my own work: *Degeneration and Regeneration in the Nervous System*, translated into English by Dr. Raoul May (Oxford University Press, London, 1928). (Cajal's 1933 footnote)

progressively increases in length. The protoplasm which surrounds the nucleus wanders toward the periphery of the ganglion.

I have found an analogous phenomenon in the granule cells of the cerebellum. At first these cells are bipolar and lie near the surface of the cerebellum. They then become monopolar while elongating and displacing their cell body as they pass through the molecular layer of the level of the deep granular layer. It is only then that the protoplasmic branches are formed.*

At this time it is probably impossible to demonstrate the chemotaxis by observations or direct experimentation. Even if it were to be considered certain, one could not assume that there is one and the same mode of growth for all nerve processes. Perhaps the following cases could be differentiated: the migration of the cell bodies themselves, the growth of axis cylinders toward certain cells, the reciprocal growth of associated nerve processes, and the growth in different directions of the protoplasmic processes and the axis cylinder of a single cell, etc.

1. The Migration of the Cell Bodies

The migration of cell bodies without a substantial change in the location of the axis cylinder can be observed in many embryonic nerve cells of the medulla and, as noted above, especially in the primordial granular layer of the cerebellum and the cell body of the sensory ganglion cells. For such cases one must assume either a *positive chemotaxis*, toward the direction in which the cells move, or a *negative chemotaxis*, which is active in the region of the axis cylinder and compels the cell to flee this axis cylinder until it happens on a mechanical barrier composed of the connective membrane of the ganglion, the bundles of the white matter in the cerebellum, etc.

2. The Growth of the Sensory and Motor Axis Cylinders

The centrifugal growth of nerve fibers to the epithelial cells, muscle fibers, etc. is very difficult to explain, even if it is as-

---

* This opinion has already been expressed by my brother, Pedro Ramón y Cajal, in his work: "El encéfalo de los reptiles." *Trabajo del laboratorio de histologia de la Universidad de Zaragoza.* 1891, p. 30. (Cajal's 1894 note)

sumed that the axis cylinder traverses over such an enormous distance because of a chemotaxis. At the outset one must suppose that both the influence of the existing barriers as well as the loci offering the least resistance are factors influencing growth (His' theory). Chemotaxis would probably become effective at a subsequent growth stage, i.e. when the nerve fibers enter that region of cells which will receive their terminal arborizations. The attracting substances would then be secreted by the epithelial, glandular, muscular, etc. cells.*

3. The Reciprocal Growth of Associated Nerve Cells

In those cells whose arborizations tend to make contact with one another and form a plexus, it would be possible to imagine *a positive reciprocal and cross-chemotaxis.* Several facts might be accounted for by this hypothesis, e.g. how the end-feet of the rods and cones manage to place themselves in contact with very specific bipolar cells, and how the arborizations of the ganglion cells come into contact exclusively with the lower clusters of certain spongioblasts.†

4. The Growth of the Nerve and Protoplasmic Processes in Different Directions

As an example of this, I will cite the Purkinje cells. Initially these cells are pyriform, and they have only a descending nerve process. They then come under the influence of an attracting

---

*After concluding this work I received a highly interesting monograph of Strasser ("Alte und neue Probleme der entwickelungsgeschichtlen Forschung auf dem Gebiet des Nervensystems," *Ergebon. d. Anat. Entwickelungsgesch.*, 1892.) The growth of nerves toward muscles and sensory organs is dealt with here. According to Strasser the cause of growth is an electromotor phenomenon. Under the influence of an electronegative condition of the myotome, the neuroblasts become excited, and their outer pole (the side of the axis cylinder) becomes electrically positive. The outgrowth of the cell body at the location of this pole (the axis cylinder) and the shift of the cell as a whole toward the muscle plate would be the result of electrical attraction in the direction of the greatest potential difference. I will return to a discussion of this hypothesis later. (1894 edition)

† By this hypothesis one would also understand the fact that protoplasmic branches of coupled elements appear simultaneously. (1892 edition)

substance which is secreted in the centers where these processes will terminate. As soon as the axis cylinder has reached its target, it becomes quiescent and is *chemotaxically indifferent*. Furthermore the cell body is the site of a positive chemotaxis for the substances produced at the level of the developing parallel fibrils which are forming in the molecular layer. The protoplasmic arborization is formed under this influence. In their direction and shape, the secondary branches retain a certain relationship to the direction and the number of the parallel fibrils.

The hypothetical role which the epithelial cells and their limiting membranes might play in this process would be to direct the amoeboid movements of the processes and to prevent them from going blindly in a straight line toward the chemotaxic source instead of following the direction most appropriate for a given anatomical structure. According to this view one may understand why the axis cylinders which arise from the retinal ganglion cells and are chemotaxically attracted toward certain elements of the brain do not deviate from their course and go into the inner part of the eye: The inner limiting membrane serves as a restraining barrier. There is no direct influence of the Müller fibers on the morphology and direction of the nerve cells themselves, since when the Müller cells send out their lamellar extensions to form the cellular pockets and the framework of the inner plexiform layer, the cell bodies and fibers of the retinal nerve cells are already completely differentiated.

This theory can also be applied to other nerve centers. Thus, in the brain, during the first stage of development the epithelial cells might exert an influence on the morphology of the pyramidal cells. Ependymal cells have an affinity for the spindle shape, as we know from the work of Magini, Falzacappa, Cajal, and Retzius. Thus, in addition to chemotaxis, the radial direction of their peripheral fibers which are inserted in the pia mater, might to some extent influence the orientation and growth of the protoplasmic trunks of the pyramidal cells toward the surface of the brain. A circumstance which also seems to support this mechanical influence is that the peripheral branches of the outer terminations of the epithelial cells have the same form and location and also appear at the same time as the terminal clusters of the peripheral trunks of the pyramidal cells (in the first cerebral layer). On the other hand, the occurrence of both the nerve and protoplasmic collaterals as well as the direction of the axis cylinder of association and commissural cells cannot be explained from the shape and orientation of the epithelial cells of the brain. Still, it is a very significant fact that the embryonic epithelial cells of the centers (in the spinal cord, Ammon's horn or hippocampus, cerebral cortex, optic lobe, etc.) always have the same orientation as the primordial nerve cell processes. What I have said already suffices to show that if in addition to the mechanical influence of the connective tissue, both inside and outside the nervous system, a chemotaxic excitability of the neuroblasts in either the positive or the negative sense is assumed, then one can begin to understand the puzzling phenomenon of the morphology of certain nerve cells and the equally mysterious fact of the contiguous relationships which are established between distant cells.

The hypothesis given here does not pretend to explain everything; it presupposes certain chemical and morphological processes for which we have no explanation at this time.* And even if the hypothesis were regarded as proven, it only clarifies certain secondary processes in the growth of the cells, while the primary conditions for the development of the cells, which are confounded with the cause of cellular change itself, are now and probably will continue to remain in total obscurity for years to come.

Nevertheless a scientific hypothesis, however weak, is better than no explanation at all. Thus, the hypothesis deserves to be provisionally accepted, despite the valid objections which could be raised. Perhaps the research which is done either to support

---

*For example, the initial distribution of epithelial cells and connective tissue which serves to check and to bar growth in certain directions; the production in different parts of the brain of attracting or repelling substances according to pre-established laws; the suspension or transformation of the chemotaxic state in each element at a predetermined time, etc. One might say that this theory ignores the difficulty without resolving it. (1892 edition)

or to refute this hypothesis will reveal facts on which to base a more solid theory of the mysterious process of the growth of nerve cells.

REFERENCES

1. Babuchin, A.: Beiträge zur Entwickelungsgeschichte des Auges, besonders der Retina. *Würzb. naturw. Zeitschr.*, 1863 (4), 71.
2. Löwe, L.: Die Histogenese der Retina nebst vergleichenden Bemerkungen über die Histogenese des Central-Nervensystems. *Arch. f. mikrosk. Anat.*, 1878 (15), 596-630.
3. Ogneff: Histogenese der Retina. *Medic. Centralbl.*, 1881, No. 35.
4. Bellonci, G.: Contribution à l'histogénèse de la couche moléculaire interne de la rétine. *Arch. ital. d. Biol.*, 1883 (3), 196-197.
5. Koganeï, Untersuchugen über die Histogenese der Retina. *Arch. f. mikrosk. Anat.*, 1884 (23), 335-357.
6. Chievitz, J.: Die Area und Fovea centralis retinae beim menschlichen Foetus. *Intern. Monatsschr. f. Anat. u. Physiol.*, 1887 (4), 201-206.
7. Kölliker, A.: *Embryologie des Menschen und der Wirbeltiere.* Leipzif, 1882, p. 717 (2nd edition).
8. His, W.: Die Neuroblasten und deren Entwickelung im embryonalen Marke. *Arch. f. Anat. u. Entwickelungsgesch.*, 1887.
9. von Lenhossék, M.: Zur Kenntnis der Entstehung der Nervenzellen und Nervenfasern beim Vogelembryo. *Arch. f. Anat. u. Physiol., Anat. Abt.*, 1890.
10. Ramón y Cajal, S.: A quelle époque apparaissent les expansions des cellules nerveuses de la moelle épinière du poulet? *Anat. Anz.*, 1890.
11. Müller, W.: Über Stammesentwicklung des Sehorgans der Wirbeltiere. *Beiträge zur Anat. u. Physiol.*, Leipzig, 1874.
12. His, W.: *Untersuchungen über die erste Anlage des Wirbeltierleibes.* Leipzig, 1868.
13. Kölliker, A.: *Embryologie des Menschen und der Wirbeltiere*, 2nd ed. Leipzig, 1882, p. 709.
14. His, W.: Zur Geschichte des menschlichen Rückenmarks und der Nervenwürzeln. *Abhandl. d. math-phys. Klasse d. K. Sächs Gesellsch. d. Wissensch.*, 1887 (13), 477.

    His, W.: Zur Geschichte des Gehirns, sowie der centralen und peripherischen Nervenbahnen beim menschlichen Embryo. *Abhandl. d. math.-phys. Klasse d. K. Sächs Gesellsch. d. Wissensch.*, 1888 (14).
15. Pfeffer, W.: Untersuchungen aus dem botanischen Institut in Tübingen. Vol. I. p. 363.
16. Massart, J., and Bordet, C.: Le chimiotaxisme des leucocytes. *Ann. d. l'Inst. Pasteur,* 1891 (5), 417-444.

17. Gabritschewsky, G.: Propriétés chimiotactiques des leucocytes. *Ann. d. l'Inst. Pasteur,* 1800 (4), 346-362.
18. Buchner, H.: Die chemische Reizbarkeit der Leukocyten und deren Beziehung zur Entsündung und Eiterung. *Berliner klin. Wochenschr.,* 1890 (6), 1084-1089.
19. Metchnikoff, I.: *Lesons sur la pathologie comparée de l'inflammation.* Paris, 1892.

Chapter X

GENERAL CONCLUSIONS

1. The nerve cells, the epithelial cells, the cones, and the rods of the retina are all completely independent elements in all vertebrates. They are true *neurons* in Waldeyer's sense.

2. The transmission of the nerve impulse from cell to cell takes place by means of articulation or contact between the various elements of the retina. Such a contact sometimes occurs only between the processes of two nearby cells; however, usually a larger number of cells make contact with one another. For example, the ascending cluster of a bipolar cell destined for the cones makes contact with several cone pedicles, and in turn each cone pedicle can contact the fibers of several bipolar cells.

3. The rods of teleost fish, nocturnal birds, and mammals have a common characteristic: They terminate with a rather roundish swelling in the outer stratum of the outer plexiform layer. On the other hand, the rods of diurnal birds and of frogs terminate with a conical foot which is covered with horizontal filaments.

4. In addition to the straight or common cones, visual cells with diagonal descending fibers are found in frogs, reptiles, and birds. Their basal swelling lies deeper than those of other visual cells.

5. In teleost fish and mammals there are two types of bipolar cell: (a) bipolars destined for the rods; their upper cluster is vertical and makes contact with the terminal spherules of the rods; and (b) bipolars destined for the cones; their upper cluster is very flat and lies in a deeper zone. The cone bipolar cell makes contact specifically with the terminal swellings and fibrils of the cones.

6. The extent of the upper terminal clusters of the bipolars destined for either the rods or the cones is quite variable. Thus, certain bipolar cells receive and transmit the excitation from a large number of visual cells whereas other bipolar cells do so for only a small number of visual cells.

7. There is a direct relation between the volume and the number of horizontal cells on the one hand and the thinness and abundance of rods on the other. Thus, in mammals and teleost fish, where the rods are very slender and quite numerous, the horizontal cells are remarkably well developed. The opposite is observed in reptiles, frogs, and birds, in which the rods are either absent (reptiles) or not very numerous.

8. According to the position and connections of the inner and outer horizontal cells, it may be surmised that they serve to bring particular groups of rods into contact with certain other groups which lie more or less distant from them. They could also have other functions which are not yet known.

9. The two types of spongioblasts described by Dogiel occur in the retinae of frogs, reptiles, and birds: (a) spongioblasts with an axis cylinder which is continuous with an optic nerve fiber,* and (b) spongioblasts without a nerve process, or amacrine cells. In mammals and teleost fish I have found only amacrine cells.

10. The amacrine cells may be placed in three classes, according to the shape of their terminal cluster: (a) cells with a flat radial cluster which seem to be composed of very long nerve fibrils, (b) cells whose cluster appears thicker and shorter, and are comprised of very gnarled, varicose protoplasmic processes, and (c) cells whose cluster has only a few thick branches which resemble protoplasmic trunks.

The first two types of amacrine cells are found in all sublayers of the inner plexiform layer. The third type, which is giant-sized, is found in only a few sublayers; these cells stain only rarely.

11. The inner plexiform layer of all vertebrates appears to be composed of four, five, or more superposed or stacked plexuses. At each of these sublayers, the terminal arborizations of the amacrine cells, the terminal clusters of the bipolar cells, and terminal arborizations of the ganglion cells interlace. The number of plexuses is always proportional to the quantity and smallness of the bipolar cells.

---

*It would have been preferable to designate these cells as spongioblasts with an axis cylinder as displaced ganglion cells, or displaced neurons. (1933 edition)

12. At present the role of the amacrine cells has not been determined; it can be said only that they must exert some influence on the clusters of the ganglion cells and perhaps also on the clusters of the bipolar cells. This effect might have its origin in the higher nerve centers and communicate with the amacrine cells by means of the terminal ramifications of the centrifugal fibers.

13. In mammals, and perhaps in all vertebrates, the inner plexiform layer contains horizontal amacrine cells at different levels.

14. In frogs, reptiles, and birds the bipolar cells often send out collateral branches to different sublayers of the inner plexiform layer. In teleost fish and mammals collateral branches are never found on the bipolar cells with ascending clusters, or those destined for the rods. It is also unusual to find collateral branches on bipolar cells destined for the cones.

15. In mammals and teleost fish the lower terminal clusters of the bipolar cells destined for the rods usually touch the upper surface of the ganglion cells.

16. The ganglion cells are constructed differently, each according to its form, extent, and also the number of sublayers in which it arborizes. The following types can be distinguished here: (a) small single-layered cells (arborizing in only one layer, "Cellules monoestratifiées") which make contact with only a few bipolar cells in the same sublayer, (b) large single-layered cells which make contact with many bipolar cells from the same sublayer, (c) large or small multilayered cells ("Cellules poliestratifiées") which transmit the activity from bipolar cells of two or three sublayers, and (d) diffuse cells ("Cellules diffuses") or diffusely ramifying cells which make contact with the bipolar cells in all or most of the sublayers. I cannot be absolutely sure if there are ganglion cells which connect exclusively with spongioblasts.

17. The lower terminal ramifications of the bipolar cells are very small, when compared with the terminal ramifications of ganglion cells. Even the smallest single-layered ganglion cells convey to the higher centers the sensations from a relatively large number of bipolar cells. Since each individual bipolar cell

receives in its turn the excitation of a large number of visual cells via its ascending cluster, it follows that *the light sensation becomes more concentrated as it proceeds through the retina.*

18. Since certain ganglion cell bodies directly receive the insertion of terminal clusters from bipolar cells destined for the rods, and since their arborizations probably also make contact with the clusters of bipolars destined for the cones, it can be assumed that these ganglion cells conduct two types of specific impulses: *the color sensation and the simple brightness sensation.* I consider it very likely that there are single-layered ganglion cells which make connection exclusively with either the bipolar cells destined for the cones or with the bipolar cells destined for the rods, so that only one of the two types of light impulses is isolated and transmitted. This point remains obscure and requires further investigation.

19. The impulse generated in the cones and in the rods is conducted in the same manner through the retina as a stimulus is conducted on all sensory surfaces, i.e. the stimulus is received by protoplasmic processes, transmitted (in a cellulifugal direction) by the axis cylinder, and fixed by the terminal ramifications of the latter process. This confirms *the law of the dynamic polarity of nerve cells* which has been formulated by van Gehuchten[1] and myself.[2] In order to apply this theory in the retina, we must consider the descending fibers of the bipolar cells as true axis cylinders and the fibers of the upper clusters as protoplasmic processes. This is an assumption which seems entirely natural, judging from the morphological characteristics of these cells. Within the retina and along the course of the visual path there are two points of branching or articulation. One is located at the level of the outer plexiform layer, and the other lies within the various sublayers of the inner plexiform layer.

The law of dynamic or functional polarity can also be applied to the spongioblasts. An impulse would be conducted to the cell body from the centrifugal fibers which originate in the higher nervous centers. Furthermore, the descending trunk of the amacrine cell and its terminal branches, despite their variegated appearance, must be regarded as functional processes. A cellulifugal current flows in these processes which then acts on the horizontal clusters of the ganglion cells.

20. From their morphological characteristics, four types of nerve cells can be distinguished in the retina: (a) neuroepithelial cells (rods and cones), (b) cells with a short nerve process (bipolar cells and horizontal cells), (c) cells with a long nerve process (ganglion cells and nervous spongioblasts), (d) amacrine cells, or those cells with no functionally differentiated process. These last elements are comparable to the granule cells of the olfactory bulb, or more so, to the monopolar cells of invertebrates (Retzius, von Lenhossék, etc.).

21. The location of individual retinal elements may vary within certain boundaries without altering their protoplasmic or nerve connections. The cell bodies which are not in their usual place are the so-called displaced cell bodies ("Cellules deplacèes"). Thus there are (a) displaced cone cell bodies (in the teleost) where the nucleus of the cone lies external to the outer limiting membrane, (b) displaced bipolars (in frogs and reptiles, etc.), (c) displaced ganglion cells (Dogiel's nervous spongioblasts, several ganglion cells in reptiles which lie within the inner plexiform layer), and (d) displaced amacrine cells (those amacrines which lie in the middle of this zone).

22. The retina of all vertebrates contains essentially identical epithelial cells (Müller structural fibers). They seem to have a role not only in supporting the nerve elements but also in isolating the cell bodies and their protoplasmic processes, so as to prevent conduction of the current in a lateral direction at the level of the outer and inner nuclear layers. The collateral branches of the epithelial cells are absent or become very fine in those layers where nervous connections are made between cells (the outer and inner plexiform layers).

23. The optic nerve, and perhaps also the layer of optic nerve fibers in the retina of all vertebrates, contains spider-like glial cells. These cells probably form a poorly conducting medium for the nervous current in the retina, just like the epithelial cells. They are always found in abundance among the nerve fibers, thereby isolating the nerve fibers from one another and preventing a longitudinal contact between them.

24. As a whole the retina is an organ whose structure shows a remarkable uniformity across all vertebrates. The structure of the retina does not appear to become perfected as one ascends the phylogenetic scale of vertebrates. There are many modifications in its structure, but these always concern the rods and cones and are appropriate to the specializations in the visual sense in each animal. There is a greater similarity between the structure of the retina of mammals with that of the teleost fish than there is between that of mammals and birds or reptiles.

25. The fovea centralis is differentiated from other parts of the retina mainly by the fact that within an equivalent area there is a greater number of cones. The cones in the fovea are much more delicate, and their basilar swellings make contact exclusively with the cluster of a single bipolar cell.

The absence of a reduction, or an insufficient reduction, in the extent of the two surfaces of nervous contact in the inner plexiform layer (the lower clusters of the bipolars on the one hand and the upper clusters of the ganglion cells on the other), coupled with the multiplicity of cones in the fovea, accounts for the modification in structure which is seen in the perifoveal region: namely, the obliqueness of the cone fibers and the processes of the bipolar cells, the considerable thickness of the inner and outer nuclear layers, etc.

REFERENCES

1. van Gehuchten, A.: La moelle épinière et le cervelet. *La Cellule*, 1891 (7), 81-122.
2. Ramón y Cajal, S.: Significación fisiológica de las expansiones protoplasmáticas y nerviosas de las células de la sustancia gris. *Rev. d. ciencas med. d. Barcelona*, 24 June, 1891.

PUBLICATIONS OF SANTIAGO RAMÓN Y CAJAL ON THE VISUAL SYSTEM

Les problèmes histophysiologiques de la rétine. XIV. *Concilium Ophtalmologicum*, 1933, Hispaniae.

Textura de la corteza visual del gato. *Trab. d. Lab. d. Inv. biol.*, (19), Nos. 1, 2, 3, October, 1921.

La desorientación inicial de las neuronas retinianas de axon corto. *Trab. d. Lab. d. Inv. biol.*, (17), Nos. 1 and 2, June, 1919.

Contribución al conocimiento de la retina y centros ópticos de los cefalópedos. *Trab. d. Lab. d. Inv. biol. d. l. University of Madrid*, (15), 1917.

Plan fundamental de la retina de los insectos. *Bol. d. l. Soc. Esp. d. Biol.*, 19 November, 1915.

Contribución al concocimiento de los centros nerviosos de los insectos. Parte I, Retina y centros ópticos (con la colaboración de don D. Sánchez). *Trab. d. Lab. d. Inv. biol.*, (13), 1915.

Nota sobre la retina de los muscidos. *Soc. Esp. d. Hist. Nat.*, January, 1910.

Nota sobre la retina de la mosca *(M. vomiforia L.) Trab d. Lab. d. Inv. Biol.*, (7), No. 4, December, 1909.

El retículo neurofibrillar en la retina. *Trab. d. Lab. d. Invest. biol.*, (3), No. 4, 1904.

Das Neurofibrillennetz der Retina. *Intern. Monatsschr. f. Anat. u. Physiol.*, (21), 1904. (Festschrift for Dr. W. Krause.)

Sobre un foco gris especial relacionado con la cinta óptica. *Trab d. Lab. d. Inv. Biol.*, (2), 1903.

Las fibras nerviosas de origen cerebral del tubérculo cuadrigémino anterior y tálamo óptico. *Trab. d. Lab. d. Inv. Biol.*, (2), 1903.

Estudios talámicos. *Trab. d. Lab. d. Inv. Biol.*, (2), 1903.

Significación del tálamo óptico y constitución de las vías sensoriales centrales. *La Clin. mod.*, Zaragoza, 1902.

Plan de estructura del tálamo óptico. *Congr. med. intern.*, Madrid, 1903.

Contribución al estudio de la vía sensitiva central y de la estructura del tálamo óptico. *Rev. trim. microgr.*, (5), 1900.

Estudios sobre la corteza cerebral humana. I Región visual. *Rev. trim. microgr.*, (1), 1899.

Apuntes para el estudio experimental de la corteza visual del cerebro humano. *Rev. ibero-amer. d. Cien. med.*, (1), March, 1899.

Estructura del quiasma óptico: teoría general de los entrecruzamientos nerviosas. *Rev. trim. microgr.*, (1), March, 1898.

Nouvelles contributions à l'etude histologique de la rétine et à la question des anastomoses des prolongements protoplasmiques. *Journ. d. l'Anat. et d. l. Physiol.*, 13 November, 1896.

Estructura de la corteza occipital de los pequeños mamíferos. *Anales d. l. Soc. d. Histor. Nat.*, (22), 1893.

La retina de los teleósteos y algunas observaciones sobre la de los vertebrados superiores. *Trab. leido a. l. Soc. d. Histor. Nat.*, 1 June, 1892.

Notas preventivas sobre la retina y gran simpático de los mamíferos. *Gaceta Sanitaria de Barcelona,* 10 December, 1891.

Pequeñas contribuciones al conocimiento del sistema nervioso. 20 August 1891. Parte III: Estructura de la retina de los reptiles y batracios.

Sur la fine structure du lobe optique des oiseaux et sur l'origine réelle des nerfs optiques. *Journ. intern. d'Anat. e. d. Physiol.*, (8), Number 9, 1891.

Sur la morphologie et les connexions des éléments de la rétine des oiseaux. *Anat. Anz.*, No. 4, 1889.

Estructura del lóbulo óptico de las aves y origen de los nervios ópticos. *Rev. trim. d. Histol. norm. y patol.*, Nos. 3 and 4, Barcelona, 1 March, 1889.

Estructura de la retina de las aves. *Rev. trim. d. Histol. norm. y patol.*, August, 1888.

Morfología y conexiones de los elementos de la retina de las aves. *Rev. trim. d. Histol norm. y patol.*, (1), May, 1888.

Sobre unos corpúsculos especiales de la retina de las aves. *Actas d. l. Soc. Esp. d. Hist. nat.*, July, 1895.

LEGENDS FOR PLATES

MOST of these figures were drawn with the Abbe camera lucida with a Zeiss objective "C." In the large figures I have drawn cells which were taken from different sections and seen in the same animal; however, they are represented as if they were seen in a single plane.

PLATE I

Figure 1. Vertical section of perch retina, *Box salpa*. A visual cell layer; B outer limiting membrane; C layer of the visual cell nuclei; D outer plexiform layer; E inner nuclear layer; F inner plexiform layer; G ganglion cell layer; H optic nerve fiber layer. a cone; b inner segment of a rod; c terminal spherule of a rod fiber; d large bipolar cell destined for the rods; e small bipolar cell destined for the cones; f end-foot of a bipolar cell destined for the rods; g lower arborization of a small bipolar cell; h large or middle-sized ganglion cell; i bipolar cell destined for the rods; j ascending cluster of such a cell (articulation of a bipolar with a rod).

Figure 2. Vertical section through the retina of *Cyprinus carpio*; double impregnation method. a external horizontal cells; b intermediate horizontal cells; c horizontal axis cylinder of an intermediate horizontal cell; d lower spherule of a rod fiber; e internal or spindle-shaped horizontal cell; f and g other cells of the same type; h fine fiber which looks like a nerve process and is continuous with a thick cell process of a spindle-shaped cell. A amacrine cells with multiple filaments which spread in the first two sublayers of the inner plexiform layer; B spongioblast or amacrine cell which sends out branches to the fifth sublayer; C voluminous amacrine cell which sends branches to the first and fourth sublayer; D amacrine cell in the inner plexiform layer whose arborizations lie in the third and fifth sublayer; E diagonal ganglion cells.

Figure 3. An amacrine cell of the perch, *Box salpa;* surface view. The radial fibrils which look like axis cylinders can be seen; they extend horizontally at the level of one of the sublayers of the inner plexiform layer.

Figure 4. Special stellate cells of the inner nuclear layer of *Box salpa*. *A* outer plexiform layer; *B* inner plexiform layer; *a, b, d* cell bodies; *e* descending processes; *f* fibrils which look like nerve processes and which ramify within the outer plexiform layer; *g* ascending nerve fibers of unknown origin; *h* lower terminations of the longest descending processes.

Figure 5. Amacrine cells or spongioblasts from the retina of *Cyprinus carpio*. *A, B* amacrine cells of the first sublayer; *C, J* amacrine cells of the second sublayer; *D, E* amacrine cells destined for the third sublayer; *H, F, O* amacrine cells of the fourth sublayer; *I, G* amacrine cells of the fifth sublayer; *M, L* diffusely-branching amacrine cells with a descending cluster whose branches accumulate especially in the fifth sublayer; *N* diffuse amacrine cells whose diagonal clusters spread mainly in the fourth and fifth sublayers.

Figure 6. Ganglion cells of the retina of *Cyprinus carpio*. *A* diffuse ganglion cell; *B* ganglion cell spreading in the fourth sublayer; *C, D, F* single-layered arborizing ganglion cells destined for the fourth sublayer; *G* multipolar amacrine cell which forms a rich plexus in the first sublayer; *H, J* single-layered ganglion cells of the third sublayer; *I, L* single-layered ganglion cells of the second sublayer; *M* giant ganglion cell destined for the first sublayer; *E* two-layered arborizing ganglion cell; *a* spongioblast which sends out collateral branches to the first sublayer and terminal branches to the fifth sublayer. (Sublayers of the inner plexiform layer are labelled: *a* first sublayer, *b* second sublayer, *c* third sublayer, *d* fourth sublayer, at the far righthand margin.)

PLATE II

Cells of the frog retina stained with chromium-silver; double-impregnation procedure.

Figure 1. *a* bipolar cell whose descending process forms three superimposed plexuses lying atop one another; *b* displaced bipolar cell; *c* bipolar cell with a single lower arborization which lies in the fifth sublayer *(g)* of the inner plexiform layer; *f* bipolar cell with a very large upper cluster; *e* brush-shaped horizontal cell; *d* bipolar cell which forms lower arborizations in the first and second sublayers; *h* centrifugal fiber (?).

Figure 2. *a* cell body of a cone; *b* cell body of a common rod; *c* cell body of a diagonal rod; c_2 cell body of diagonal rod whose descending fiber terminates as a point with no terminal swelling; *d* very long fiber arising from a diagonal rod; *f* displaced bipolar cell; *g* Landolt club; *h* large or outer bipolar cell; *i* bipolar cell with three lower arborizations; *j* large bipolar cell; *r* diffuse spongioblast; *s* Dogiel's nervous spongioblast; *k* bipolar cell with two lower arborizations; *t* bipolar cell whose lower arborizations fill two sublayers.

Figure 3. *a* cell body of a very thick cone; *b* cell body of a rod; *c* cell body of a club-shaped rod; *d* double rod; *e* small horizontal cell; *f* fiber resembling an axis cylinder; *g* large horizontal cell with finger-like branches; *h, i* ascending fibrils which ramify in the outer plexiform layer; *j* large or outer bipolar cell. A amacrine cell destined for the first sublayer; B nervous spongioblast; C, E stellate amacrine cells destined for the second sublayer; D amacrine cell with a tangled cluster destined for the second sublayer; F, H amacrine cells of the third sublayer; L, N amacrine cells of the fourth sublayer; M amacrine cell of the fifth sublayer; O, J diffuse amacrine cells; G amacrine cell ramifying in two layers (two-layered amacrine cell).

Figure 4. *a* multilayered ganglion cell; *b, f* ganglion cells destined for the second sublayer; *d* ganglion cell destined for the first sublayer; *c* ganglion cell with a diffuse and very delicate cluster; *g* stellate fibrils which extend into two layers, perhaps originating from a ganglion cell; *h* descending fibrillar radial division of a protoplasmic trunk, probably arising from a stellate amacrine cell.

Figure 5. *a* inner segment of a common rod; *b* outer segment with black transverse striations; *c* inner segment of a cone; *d* club-shaped rod with a filiform pedicle; *e* club-shaped rod with a thicker conical foot and whose nucleus *(h)* lies below the outer limiting membrane; *i* cone nucleus; *f* nucleus of a common rod; *g* nucleus of a club-shaped rod.

Figure 6. Ganglion cells. *a* giant cell which arborizes in the second sublayer; *b* ganglion cell with a diffuse cluster; *c* giant ganglion cell which arborizes in two layers (the second and fourth sublayers); *d* three-layered ganglion cell; middle-sized *(g)* and small *(f)* two-layered ganglion cells; *e* ganglion cell with a granular cluster destined for the fourth sublayer; *h* and *k* nerve fibers which appear to penetrate the inner plexiform layer. *A* inner plexiform layer; *B* ganglion cell layer.

PLATE III

All figures in Plate III represent cells from the retina of the green lizard, *Lacerta viridis*.

Figure 1. Transverse section through a retina stained by the Golgi method (double-impregnation method). *a* cell body of a cone which lies next to the outer limiting membrane; *b* elongated cell body which lies in the intermediate region of the outer nuclear layer; *c* diagonal fiber of a cone; *d* double cone; *e* cell body of a cone with pale transverse striations; *p* outer or large bipolar cell; *o* inner or small bipolar cell; *s* Landolt club; *r* descending process of a bipolar cell with collateral branches; *q* a terminal arborization which lies above the ganglion cells; *x* fine horizontal fiber from a horizontal cell; *y* bifurcating descending process of a bipolar cell.

Figure 2. Terminal swellings of a descending cone fiber seen from their lower surface (horizontal section).

Figure 3. Transverse section through a retina stained with Grenarcher carmine. *a* cone layer; *b* cone nuclei; *c* cell bodies of displaced bipolar cells; *d* terminal swellings of the cones; *e* brush-shaped horizontal cell; *f* giant amacrine cell; *g, h, i, j* sublayers of the inner plexiform layer which appear more granulated than the rest; the second (*g*) and the third (*h*) sublayers are more developed than the others; *s, t* cell bodies which probably belong to displaced amacrine cells; *k* ganglion cell layer; *r* optic nerve fiber layer.

Figure 4. Inner plexiform layer and amacrine cells. *a* unstratified arborizing amacrine cell; *b* stellate amacrine cell which arborizes in the third sublayer; *c* amacrine cell with a twisted cluster destined for the fifth sublayer; *d* smaller amacrine cell arborizing in the fourth sublayer; *e* giant amacrine cell destined for the second sublayer, characterized by an initially thick branch which gradually becomes finer until it has the appearance of an axis cylinder (*m*); *f* stellate amacrine cell of the first sublayer; *g* stellate amacrine cell destined for the third sublayer; *h* amacrine cell with radiating cluster destined for the fourth sublayer; *i* unstratified amacrine cell with multiple processes; *k* displaced ganglion cell; *m* a fine nerve fiber arising from a giant amacrine cell (*e*).

Figure 5. *a* unstratified amacrine cell; *b, c* amacrine cells with tangled clusters destined for the second sublayer; *d* stellate amacrine cell destined for the fifth sublayer; *e* nervous spongioblast; *f* large amacrine cell destined for the third sublayer; *g* amacrine cell whose fine branches appear to spread in the first and fifth sublayers; *h* stellate amacrine cell of the second sublayer; *A, B* two ganglion cells with exceptionally fine and well developed clusters; *C* ganglion cell destined for the fourth sublayer; *D* ganglion cell whose fine ascending branches go to the first sublayer.

Figure 6. Ganglion cells of various types. A giant ganglion cell with a diffuse ramification; *B* horizontal ganglion cell, most of whose branches are distributed in the fifth sublayer; *C* multilayered ganglion cell which forms plexuses in the second, third, and fourth sublayers; *D, F* two ganglion cells with granular clusters destined for the fourth sublayer; *E* ganglion cell with a delicate cluster that fills the third, fourth, and the upper half of the fifth sublayers; *G* ganglion cell whose branches extend to the first sublayer; *H* another ganglion cell similar to cell *C* but of smaller dimensions; *I* giant ganglion cell of the second sublayer.

Figure 7. *f, h, i, g* different types of displaced bipolar cells; *j* brush-shaped horizontal cell with a fine axis cylinder; *m* stellate horizontal cell with an axis cylinder *(k)* (this cell was stained with methylene blue); *n* mitral spongioblast of large dimensions (also stained with methylene blue); *t* collateral fibrils of an optic nerve fiber from the retina of a *Lacerta agilis* embryo.

PLATE IV

Figure 1. Stellate amacrine cells from the retina of the lizard, as seen in a horizontal section through the inner plexiform layer. *a* pyriform cell body; *b* granular end of a stellate branch.

Figure 2. Giant amacrine cell from a horizontal section of the lizard retina. *a* cell body; *b* fine branches which resemble axis cylinders. The cell is of the same type as that shown in Plate III, Figure 4, *e*.

Figure 3. Surface view of a ganglion cell in the lizard as seen in a horizontal section through the retina. *a* cell body; *b* varicose branches which end freely; *c* axis cylinder which is continuous with a fiber of the optic nerve fiber layer.

Figure 4. Basilar fibrils which arise from the terminal swellings of visual cell bodies seen in a horizontal section through the chicken retina. *a* lower view of a cone terminal swelling; *b* lower view of a rod terminal swelling.

Figure 5. Brush-shaped horizontal cell from the chicken retina, as seen in a horizontal section. *a* cell body and protoplasmic processes; *b* horizontal axis cylinder; *c* terminal ramification.

Figure 6. Visual cells and horizontal cells from the turkey retina. *a* cone with a very long descending and oblique fiber; *e* collateral branches of this fiber; *b* straight cones; *c* rods; *d* double cones; *f*, *g* flat horizontal cells; *h* brush-shaped horizontal cell; *j* terminal ramification of an axis cylinder.

Figure 7. Flat horizontal cells in a horizontal section through the chicken retina. *a* cells; *b* axis cylinders.

Figure 8. Nerve cells from the chicken retina. *a* rod; *b* straight cone; *c* diagonal cone; *d* a cone whose terminal swelling lies below the outer plexiform layer; *e*, *f* double cones; *h* cone with basilar fibrils which descend in bundles; *i* brush-shaped horizontal cells; *j* flat horizontal cells; *g* terminal arborization of an axis cylinder which arises from a brush-shaped horizontal cell; *k* another similar terminal swelling; *o*, *p*, *q* thin bipolars; *l* Landolt club; *m* bipolar cell with a Landolt club; *n* thick or outer bipolar cell; *r*, *s* terminal arborizations of bipolar cells; *t* terminal arborization which extends into two adjacent sublayers. *A* small amacrine cell destined for the first sublayer; *B* same type of amacrine cell but much smaller; *C* another larger amacrine cell; *D, F* amacrine cells with dense clusters which are distributed within the second sublayer; *E* stellate amacrine cell destined for the second sublayer; *K, J* amacrine cells with twisted clusters destined for the third sublayer; *M* giant amacrine cell destined for the third sublayer; *N, H* amacrine cells destined for the fourth sublayer; *I* stellate amacrine cell of the fifth sublayer; *G, L* unstratified amacrine cells. (The numbers on the left side designate the sublayers of the inner plexiform layer.)

Figure 9. Visual cells from the retina of the green finch. *a* rod; *b* cone whose terminal swelling lies in the outer half of the outer plexiform layer; *c* cone whose swelling lies in a deeper layer; *d* diagonal cone; *e* fibrillar cluster of a rod.

Figure 10. Visual cells and bipolar cells from the retina of the green finch. *a* rod; *b* cone whose terminal swelling contacts the upper cluster of a bipolar cell; *d* bipolar cell with a flat cluster; *c* bipolar cell with a larger cluster whose fibers ascend to the level of the rod terminal swellings.

PLATE V

All figures show cells from the mammalian retina with the exception of Figure 1, which shows nerve cells from the chicken retina.

Figure 1. A ganglion cell destined for the first sublayer; B ganglion cell destined for the second sublayer; C small ganglion cells with granular clusters which spread in the fourth sublayer; D multipolar cell destined for the second sublayer; E a cell which forms two horizontal plexuses—one below the fourth sublayer and another in the third sublayer; F small cell with two fine plexuses—one in the second sublayer and the other in the fourth sublayer; G giant cell which forms three plexuses—in the second, third, and fourth sublayers; H bistratified amacrine cell; J cell with an extremely fine plexus destined for the third sublayer; K cell which arborizes in the fourth sublayer and whose branches interlace with the end branches of an amacrine cell lying in the same layer; a centrifugal fibers; b another centrifugal fiber whose termination extends horizontally above the inner plexiform layer.

Figure 2. A section through the retina of an adult dog. a cone fiber; b cell body and fiber of a rod; c bipolar cell with an ascending cluster destined for the rods; d very small bipolar cell for the rods with a sparse upper cluster; e bipolar cell with a flat cluster destined for the cones; f giant bipolar cell with a flat cluster; h diffuse amacrine cell whose varicose branches lie, for the most part, just above the ganglion cells; i ascending nerve fibrils; j centrifugal fibers; g special cells which are very rarely impregnated; they have an ascending axis cylinder; n ganglion cell which receives the terminal cluster of a bipolar cell destined for the rods; m nerve fiber which disappears in the inner plexiform layer; p nerve fiber of the optic fiber layer. A outer plexiform layer; B inner plexiform layer.

Figure 3. Horizontal cells from the adult dog retina. A outer horizontal cell; B middle-sized inner horizontal cell with no descending protoplasmic processes; C another, smaller inner horizontal cell; a horizontal axis cylinder.

Figure 4. Nerve cells from the ox retina. a bipolar cell with an ascending cluster; *b* bipolar cell with a flat upper terminal cluster destined for the cones; *c, d, e* bipolar cells of the same type whose lower cluster, however, arborizes in the more external sublayers of the inner plexiform layer; *g* bipolar cell with a flat cluster of enormous extent; *f* another bipolar cell with a giant upper cluster characterized by the rich and irregular arborization formed by the ascending process; *h* oval cells lying outside the outer plexiform layer; *i* amacrine cell located within the second sublayer of the inner plexiform layer; *j* amacrine cell occupying the third sublayer; *m* another amacrine cell whose branches apparently disappear in the third and fourth sublayers.

Figure 5. Horizontal axis cylinder from the outer plexiform layer. *a* terminal arborization as seen from the side; *b* nerve fiber.

Figure 6. Another terminal arborization of the same type.

Figure 7. Nerve elements from the ox retina stained with chromium-silver according to the double impregnation method. A semilunar amacrine cell whose enormously long branches arborize in the first sublayer; *B* large amacrine cell with thick branches in the second sublayer; *F* another amacrine cell which is rather small and arborizes in the second sublayer; *D* amacrine cell with a stellate cluster destined for the third sublayer; *G, H* amacrine cells destined for the fourth sublayer; *E* large amacrine cell destined for the fifth sublayer; *C* special type of amacrine cell with very thin branches which spread preferentially in the first and fifth sublayers. *a* small ganglion cell destined for the fourth sublayer; *b* ganglion cell whose branches form three superimposed plexuses; *c* small ganglion cell with branches arborizing in the first sublayer; *d* middle-sized ganglion cell with branches in the fourth sublayer; *f* ganglion cell which is similar to the multilayered cells (branching in three sublayers) in the reptile and bird; their branches form two plexuses—one in the fourth sublayer and another in the second sublayer; *e* giant ganglion cell destined for the third sublayer.

Figure 8. Amacrine cells and ganglion cells from the dog retina. *A* stellate amacrine cell destined for the first sublayer and a portion of the second sublayer; *B* giant amacrine cell of the third sublayer; *G, C* stellate amacrine cells destined for the second sublayer; *F* small amacrine cell destined for the third sublayer; *E* amacrine cell destined for the fourth sublayer; *D* unstratified amacrine cell; *a* ganglion cell whose upper cluster spreads in the second sublayer; *b* giant ganglion cell destined for the fifth sublayer; *e* small ganglion cell whose cluster spreads in the fourth sublayer; *f* middle-sized ganglion cell which arborizes in the first and in a portion of the second sublayers; *g* ganglion cell which arborizes in the third and a portion of the fourth sublayers; *i* two-layered cell ("Cellule bistratifée").

Figure 9. Ganglion cells from the dog retina. *a* giant ganglion cell whose cluster spreads in the first and a portion of the second sublayer; *b* small ganglion cell whose multiple processes disappear in the fifth sublayer; *c* giant cell whose cluster seems to spread mainly in the second sublayer; *e* giant ganglion cell of the second sublayer; *d, g* small ganglion cells with clusters in the fourth sublayer; *f* middle-sized ganglion cell destined for the first sublayer; *h* another ganglion cell destined for the second and partially for the first sublayer; *i* unstratified ganglion cell; *A, B, C* spongioblasts; *L* lower terminal arborization of a bipolar cell.

PLATE VI

Figure 1. Epithelial cells (or Müller supporting fibers) from the frog retina. *a* outer nuclear layer; *b* outer plexiform layer; *c* inner nuclear layer; *e* inner plexiform layer; *d* spongioblast and descending processes accompanying them; *f* ganglion cell layer; *g* basal layer or inner limiting membrane.

Figure 2. Epithelial (Müller supporting fibers) from the retina of *Cyprinus carpio*.

Figure 3. Epithelial cells from the lizard retina.

Figure 4. Epithelial cells from the chicken retina.

Figure 5. Epithelial cells from the ox retina, probably from the peripheral region. *a* descending collateral branches; *b* region of the nucleus.

Figure 6. Epithelial cells from the ox retina, probably from the region near the optic disk.

Figure 7. Horizontal axis cylinder from the plexiform layer of the ox. *a* trunk; *b* extensive varicose terminal arborization.

Figure 8. Terminal arborization of a horizontal fiber from the outer plexiform layer of the dog.

Figure 9. Another terminal arborization of the same type but from the retina of a young rabbit.

Figure 10. Terminal arborization of a very thick axis cylinder from the ox retina, seen in profile on a thick transverse section through the retina.

Figure 11. Outer horizontal cell of the ox retina seen from a horizontal section of the retina. *a* nerve fibers; *b* protoplasmic branches.

Figure 12. A vertical section through the ox retina. *a* inner horizontal cell with a descending process; *b* another cell of the same type but with no lower process; *c* mitral-shaped amacrine cell with two branches extending in opposite directions; *d* large amacrine cell destined for the fourth sublayer; *e* small ganglion cell which arborizes in the second sublayer; *f, g, h, i, j* different types of neuroglial cells; *k* interstitial amacrine cell which arborizes preferentially in two sublayers (bistratified).

Figure 13. Inner horizontal cell with no descending process, seen on a horizontal section through the ox retina. *a* horizontal axis cylinder; *b* finger-like protoplasmic branches.

Figure 14. An inner horizontal cell with a very stout descending process. *a* a nerve fiber (?).

Figure 15. Perpendicular section through the chameleon retina at the level of the fovea centralis. *a* thin cones; *b* thicker cones; *c* cell body of a cone; *e* small upper cluster of a bipolar cell; *f* amacrine cells; *g* collateral branch of an epithelial (Müller) cell.

Figure 16. Vertical section through the retina of the green finch in the area of the fovea centralis. *a* thin cones; *b* thicker cones; *e* cell body of a cone; *d* diagonal cone fiber; *c* nodosity of the cone fiber; *f* terminal swellings of the same fiber; *g* tiny cluster of a bipolar cell; *i* stratified amacrine cell; *j* ganglion cell destined for the fourth sublayer; *l* ganglion cells of the second sublayer; *h* bipolar cell in the more peripheral portion of the retina and oriented obliquely.

PLATE VII

Figure 1. Section through the retina of a mouse embryo 15 mm in length. *a* ganglion cell (neuroblast of His) which still has no protoplasmic processes; *b* a somewhat more developed cell; *c* ganglion cell with ascending and descending protoplasmic processes (*g*); *d* epithelial (Müller) cell; *e* epithelial cell whose cell body lies near the outer limiting membrane and appears to be ready to branch; *f* club-shaped cell (cell body of a rod).

Figure 2. Section through the retina of a dog embryo 9 cm in length. *a* epithelial cells; *b* bipolar cells; *g* cell bodies of the visual cells; *e* ganglion cells; *f* descending process of a Müller cell which appears to bifurcate; *n* neuroglial cell.

Figure 3. Transverse section through the retina of a fourteen-day-old chick embryo. *a* epithelial (Müller) cells; *b* inner surface of these cells, still with no ascending fibers; *c* cell body of a rod; *d* inner nuclei; *e* diagonal cone; *f* Landolt club; *m* bipolar cell; *n* straight cone; *s* pyriform amacrine cell; *u* giant amacrine cell; *t* multilayered ganglion cell.

Figure 4. Horizontal (anteroposterior) section through the eye of a mouse embryo 15 mm in length. A anterior epithelium of the crystalline lens; B prisms of the lens; C retinal fold; *a* layer of optic fibers; *b* epithelial cells; *c* ganglion cell.

Figure 5. Inner horizontal cells from the ox retina. A, C fusiform cells; B stellate cell with a very long horizontal process which arborizes in the inner plexiform zone (*a*).

Figure 6. Several outer horizontal cells with a descending process, taken from the ox retina. *a* cell with descending processes which arborize extensively in a horizontal orientation; *b* much smaller cell of the same type; *c* cell whose axis cylinder can be traced over a great extent; *d* much smaller cell with a single descending process which arborizes within a small area.

Figure 7. Outer horizontal cell from the ox retina seen on an oblique section. *a* axis cylinder which gives off collateral branches.

Figure 8. Nerve cells from an ox retina stained with methylene blue (the Ehrlich-Dogiel method). *a* bipolar cells destined for the cones; *b* giant bipolar cell with a flat cluster; *c* bipolar

Legends for Plates

cell destined for the cones; the cell body lies near the inner plexiform layer; *d* semilunar spongioblasts with very fine, long branches which disappear mostly in the fifth sublayer; *f* diffuse amacrine cells which are often stained with methylene blue; they form a very dense, granular plexus *(g)* in the fifth sublayer; *e* pyriform amacrine cells destined for the third sublayer; *h* amacrine cell of the first sublayer; *i* amacrine cell destined for the second sublayer; *j* triangular amacrine cell lying within the fourth sublayer; *k* giant ganglion cell whose body exhibits granules which are stained very intensely with methylene blue; *m* ganglion cell without such granules and which apparently spreads in the third sublayer.

Figure 9. Outer or small horizontal cells of an ox retina stained with methylene blue. *a* cell body with very intense blue flecks; *b* very fine and extensively branched protoplasmic processes; *c* axis cylinders on which it is impossible to see collateral branches; *d* thicker axis cylinders which sometimes arborize and probably originate from the large or inner horizontal cells.

Figure 10. Outer horizontal cell from the sheep retina seen in a diagonal section. *a* ramified axis cylinder.

Figure 11. Amacrine cells from the retina of a two-day-old rabbit. *a* amacrine cell of the first sublayer; *b* amacrine cell probably destined for the third sublayer.

Figure 12. Nerve cells from the retina of a two-day-old rabbit. *a* club-shaped cells; *b* rods; *c* inner horizontal cell with a descending process; *d* horizontal cell without descending processes.

IV

NAME INDEX

Angelucci, 39
Apáthy, 12

Babuchin, 140, 145
Baquis, xxx, xxxv, 7, 30, 93, 95, 101, 105, 125
Beauregard, 76
Bellonci, 140
Boll, 4, 39
Bordet, 146
Borysiekiewicz, 4, 33, 93, 119, 128
Buchner, 146

Chiewitz, 134, 140, 145
Corti, xxvi, 124

Denissenko, 17
Dobrowsky, 76
Dogiel, xiii, xviii, xxviii, xxix, xxxiv, 5, 6, 7, 11, 12, 20, 30, 31, 42, 44, 45, 46, 47, 48, 51, 64, 66, 82, 89, 90, 91, 93, 95, 97, 98, 99, 101, 102, 104, 105, 106, 110, 111, 112, 113, 114, 119, 125

Edinger, xv, xxxiv
Ehrlich, xv, xviii
Ewald, 39

Falzacappa, 149
Forel, xxv, 12
Fromaget, xxx

Gabritschewsky, 146
Gerlach, xxiv
Golgi, xi, xv, xvi, xviii, xxiii, xxix, 4, 33, 97, 128, 129

Hannover, 4, 17
Held, 143

Henle, xxvi
His, xi, xvi, xxv, xxxi, xxxiv, 7, 12, 142, 148
Hoffmann, 40, 47, 60, 62, 76, 79

Jones, xxvi

Kallius, xxii, xxxi
Koganeï, 140
Kölliker, xi, xv, xvi, xxxiv, 4, 12, 97, 142, 143, 145
Krause, 11, 17, 20, 21, 22, 23, 24, 40, 42, 44, 45, 76, 93, 97, 125, 126, 134, 136
Kühne, 4, 39
Kuhnt, 4, 93, 134

Landolt, 47
Leber, 129
Lenox, 93
Löwe, 140

Magini, 149
Manfredi, 33, 97, 128, 129
Massart, 146
Merkel, xxxi, xxxiv, xxxv, xxxvi, 97
Metchnikoff, 146
Monakow, 89
Müller, H., xxvii, 4, 20, 33, 119, 133, 134
Müller, W., 4, 17, 142, 143

Nagel, 33, 119
Nicati, 54

Ogneff, 140

Petrone, 129
Pfeffer, 146

Ranvier, 4, 17, 30, 42, 45, 47, 58, 60, 62, 93, 97, 124, 125
Reich, 17, 22
Retzius, xvi, xviii, xxx, xxxiv, 7, 12, 13, 17, 113, 149
Riese, xvi
Ritter, 33
Rivolta, 4, 97, 98

Sala, xxxiv
Schiefferdecker, 4, 20, 21, 22, 23, 24, 42, 45, 75, 80, 93, 97, 98
Schultze, xxvii, 4, 17, 23, 40, 60, 76, 79, 94, 134

Schwalbe, xxxi, 4, 17, 21, 22, 23, 40, 58, 76, 93, 97, 128, 129
Sömmering, xxvi
Strasser, 148

Tartuferi, xi, xxviii, xxix, xxxi, xxxv, 5, 6, 7, 11, 46, 93, 94, 95, 98, 99, 100, 101, 102, 105, 106, 110, 111, 126
Tello, 143

van Gehuchten, xvi, xxxiv, 7, 12, 13
von Lenhossék, xvi, xix, xxxiv, 12, 113, 142

Waldeyer, xi, xvi, xxxiv

SUBJECT INDEX

A

Amacrine cells, xxxiii, 19, 29, 153, 155, 157
  as neuroglia, 84
  bird retina, 83-87, 89
  bistratified, 33, 50, 51, 70, 118, 120
  development of, 143, 145
  diffuse, 30, 49, 67, 83, 116
  displaced, 52, 115, 119, 120
  fish retina, 29-33
  frog retina, 48-51
  in fovea, 135, 137, 138
  mammalian retina, 111-120
  monostratified, 30-33, 49-50, 67-70, 84-85
  reptile retina, 66-70

B

Bipolar cells, xxviii, 5, 6, 109, 153, 155, 157
  bird retina, 82-83
  cone bipolar cells, xxxi, 7, 8, 25, 26, 46, 66, 80, 96, 97, 108, 109, 153
  development of, 143, 144
  displaced, 6, 42, 43, 60, 62, 79, 115
  fish retina, 24-27
  frog retina, 45-48
  in fovea, 134, 135, 136, 137
  inner (small) bipolar cells, 26-27, 46-47, 64-65
  mammalian retina, 106-111
  outer (large) bipolar cells, 25-26, 45-46, 65-66
  reptile retina, 64-66
  rod bipolar cells, xxxi, 7, 8, 25, 26, 46, 80, 96, 107, 108, 153
Bird retina, 3, 20, 24, 26, 28, 31, 42, 57, 63, 64, 76-92, 93, 95, 109, 114, 115, 116, 121, 122, 133, 134, 135, 145

C

Calf retina, 140
Cat retina, 93, 98, 103, 104
Centrifugal fibers, 6, 57, 74, 85, 86, 87, 89, 90, 126, 127, 145, 155
Cerebellum, xvii, xxii, 3
  granule cells, 147
  Purkinje cells, xxii, xxiii, 91, 148
Cerebral cortex, 150
Chameleon retina, 60, 135, 136, 137, 138
Chicken retina, 90, 140, 141, 143, 145
Chromium-silver stain, see Golgi method
Cones, xxxii, 6, 8, 153, 157
  bird retina, 76, 80
  development of, 144, 145
  diagonal cones, 61, 77-79
    in bird retina, 77-79
    in reptile retina, 61
  fish retina, 19
  frog retina, 39, 41, 42
  in fovea, 133, 136
  mammalian retina, 94-96
  straight cones, 60, 61, 77
    in bird retina, 77
    in reptile retina, 60, 61
  transmission of cone signals, 27, 109, 110
Cyprinids, 12, 23, 28

D

Development of retinal cells, 140-152
  amacrine cells, 143
  bipolar cells, 143, 144
  centrifugal fibers, 145
  epithelial cells, 140, 141
  ganglion cells, 141
  horizontal cells, 145
  Landolt clubs, 143, 144
  optic nerve, 141, 142

photoreceptors, 144, 145
Displaced retinal cells, 6, 115, 157
Dog retina, 93, 98, 103, 104, 105, 118, 120, 126
Double cones
  bird retina, 78, 79
  frog retina, 42, 79
  reptile retina, 60, 61, 78, 79
  significance, 79
Double rods, 42

E

Ehrlich method, *see* Methylene blue

F

Finch retina, 77, 81, 86, 88, 89, 133
Fish retina, *see* Teleost fish retina
Fovea centralis, 133-139, 158
  in chameleon, 135-138
  in sparrow, 133-135
  "private path," 135, 138
Frog retina, 26, 28, 39-59, 64, 79, 85, 87, 88, 109, 112, 114, 125, 145

G

Ganglion cells, xxxi, xxxii, xxxiii, 55, 126, 155, 157
  bird retina, 87-89
  bistratified, 36, 53, 54, 72, 88, 122, 123
  development of, 141, 142, 145
  diffuse, 36, 54, 73, 123, 124
  displaced, 73, 120
  fish retina, 34-36
  frog retina, 52-54
  in fovea, 135, 137, 138
  mammalian retina, 120-126
  monostratified, 35-36, 52, 53, 70-72, 87-88, 120-122
  multistratified, 36, 54, 72-73, 88, 122-123
  reptile retina, 70-74
Golgi method, xi, xii, xv, xvii, xxvii, 4, 5, 11, 114

characteristics, xvii, xxiii
comparison with methylene blue stain, xvii, xviii, xxxv, 47, 90
counter-staining, 15
eye size, 13
results, xviii, xxii, xxiii, xxiv
rolling-up procedure, 14, 15
technique, xix, xx, xxii, xxiii, 12, 13

H

Hippocampus, 150
Horizontal cells, xxxiii, 20, 43, 153, 157
  as glial cells, 23
  bird retina, 81-82
  contact with photoreceptors, 21, 24, 44, 64, 81, 100, 103
  development of, 145
  fish retina, 20-24
  frog retina, 43-45
  inner horizontal cells, 22, 23, 24, 44, 45, 101, 102, 104
  intermediate horizontal cells, 21, 22
  mammalian retina, 97-102
  as nerve cells, 22, 45
  outer horizontal cells, 20, 43, 44, 99, 100
  reptile retina, 63, 64
Horse retina, 93
Human retina, 22, 95, 110, 112, 113, 139

I

Inner plexiform layer, xxxiii, 29, 30, 31, 57, 66, 74, 89, 105, 110, 112, 124, 125, 153

L

Landolt clubs, 5, 106
  bird retina, 82, 106
  development of, 143, 144
  frog retina, 43, 47, 106
  in fovea, 134
  mammalian retina, 106
  reptile retina, 62, 64, 106

Lens, 143
Lizard retina, 60, 62, 141

M

Mammalian retina, 24, 28, 55, 57, 80, 85, 87, 88, 93-132, 145
Medulla, xxiv, 147
Mouse retina, 93, 140
Müller cell, 5, 17, 157
  bird retina, 91
  development of, 140, 141
  fish retina, 37
  frog retina, 58
  function, 58, 149, 150
  in fovea, 138
  mammalian retina, 127, 128
  reptile retina, 74, 75

N

Nerve net, xxiv, xxv, xxvi, xxviii, xxx, xxxiv, xxxv, 3, 46, 90, 95, 110, 125
Neural contact, xxv, xxix, xxx, xxxi, xxxiv, xxxv, 3, 90, 153
Neural growth theories, 142, 146, 147, 148, 149, 150
Neuroblast, 29, 142
Neuroglia, xxxi, 27, 28, 37, 57, 74, 91, 127, 128, 129, 130, 137, 157

O

Oil droplets, 76, 79
Olfactory bulb, 3, 29
Olfactory mucosa, 143
Optic nerve, 157
  bird retina, 89
  development of, 141-142
  fish retina, 37
  frog retina, 54-57
  frog retina, 42, 56-57
  mammalian retina, 126-127
  reptile retina, 74
Outer plexiform layer
  bird retina, 80-81
  fish retina, 19-20
  mammalian retina, 97, 102-105
  reptile retina, 61-62
Ox retina, 93, 97, 99, 103, 104, 105, 119
Owl retina, 80

P

Perch retina, 17, 23, 28
Pig retina, 93, 98
Pigeon retina, 86, 90
Pigment migration, 39

R

Rabbit retina, 98, 104, 140, 145
Reptile retina, 26, 28, 42, 60-75, 79, 83, 85, 87, 88, 109, 110, 112, 115, 120, 121, 122
Retinal organization, xxxi, xxxii, 3, 4, 27, 85-87, 109-110, 124, 125, 135, 138, 139, 156, 158
Rods, xxxi, 6, 7, 8, 153, 157
  bird retina, 76, 77, 80
  development of, 144, 145
  fish retina, 18, 19
  green rods, 40, 41, 42
  mammalian retina, 94-96
  photopigment in, 23
  red rods, 39-42
  reptile retina, 60
  transmission of rod signals, 27, 109, 110

S

Salamander retina, 39, 47
Sheep retina, 93, 98, 105
Sparrow retina, 77, 81, 85, 88, 90, 133, 134, 135
Spinal cord, xviii, xxiv, 3, 142, 146, 147, 150
Spongioblasts, 28, 126, 153, 157
  bird retina, 90
  development of, 143, 145

fish retina, 28
frog retina, 48, 51
mammalian retina, 111
reptile retina, 66
Staining techniques, *see* Golgi method, methylene blue
   carmine, xv, 3
   Cox, 11, 125
   hematoxylin, xv
   osmic acid, 3
   Weigert, xxxv

T

Terminology, v, xiii, 17, 18
Teleost fish retina, 17-38, 55, 87, 88, 93, 105, 109, 126
Tortoise retina, 62
Turkey retina, 78